Attention Educators

The following instructional aids complement *Anyone Can Intubate* and are available from the publisher. See **page 239** for details.

Teacher's Guide — Chapter by chapter teaching suggestions and multiple-choice k-style tests, **free** to adopting institutions.

Slides: color graphics on Intubation and Airway Management.

Videos: Basic Intubation, Managing the Airway, Pediatric Airway Management and Intubation, Nasotracheal Intubation, Fiberoptic Intubation

CEU credit — Available through Kaiser Permanente, Nursing Education Office. You do not have to be a resident of California to receive this credit. Write or call **619-528-6133** for details.

What readers and reviewers said about earlier editions of *Anyone Can Intubate:*

British Journal of Anaesthesia
". . . a superb handbook for those needing to acquire the skills of tracheal intubation and I shall certainly include it in our basic instruction system for medical undergraduates . . . Dr. Whitten takes us through well illustrated airway anatomy, equipment, techniques and complications. She includes a sensible discussion on general airway management and basic ventilation, leading eventually to the handling of the crisis situation by needle crico-thyrotomy. The sections on common errors and difficult intubations are most valuable for the trainee. The line drawings are well placed within the text and are a prime asset of the book." **— T. Hilary Howells**

Anesthesiology
"Individuals charged with the task of teaching airway management will benefit from reading the author's step-by-step approach to teaching the complex psychomotor skill of laryngoscopy and may apply many principles found in the text in their own airway instruction. The author is to be credited for this important effort to provide young health professionals a thoughtful approach to learning (and teaching) lthis often difficult but lifessaving skill." **— Frederick W. Campbell, MD**

Critical Care Nurse
". . . accurate, easy to read, and clearly illustrated." **— Irene Grossback, RN, MS**

Adopted by the **Nurse's Book Society**.

Serialized in *Emergency Medicine* magazine.

— over for more reviews –

Postgraduate Medicine

"I heartily recommend *Anyone Can Intubate* for all health-care personnel who in their daily activities are "at risk" for code participating. This book will go far in renewing their confidence in a necessary skill." — **Donald E. DeWitt, MD**

Annals of Emergency Medicine

"This book is an easy read, with a relaxed tone and style. *Anyone Can Intubate* is a potentially valuable resource for paramedic and medical students.."
— **Daniel F. Danzl, MD, FACEP**

AORN Journal

"During the 10 or more years that the American Heart Association has sponsored advanced cardiac life support training, I do not recall seeing such a systematic and concise account of intubation . . . detailed instruction that is sorely needed in the apprenticeship of life support. This discussion is extremely valuable. Overall, the text is well worth its price." — **Marian Shaughnessey, RN, MSN, CNOR**

I found the text to be informative, easy to read, and should provide the reader with a sound basis when learning how to intubate. The illustrations contribute greatly to the text. They are superb! The chapters addressing the difficult airway and intubation contain much practical information often overlooked when teaching intubation techniques. They really make the book a complete guide to intubation. The textbook fills in all the gaps in intubation instruction and should benefit anyone who needs to learn how to intubate." — **Thomas G. Healey, CRNA, MA**
V.P., American Association of Nurse Anesthetists

"Excellent illustrations. Concise presentation of material." — **Allen Barbaro**
Program Director, Respiratory Care
Odessa College, Texas

Kaiser Permanente, Southern California Region

"The staff and I have reviewed the book and find the format and presentation of information offered in a very direct and understandable manner. The content is outstanding as to objectives and visual aids (figures). We will use it for our class presentation and as a student resource." — **Joyce W. Kelly, CRNA, MA**
Dir., School of Anesthesia for Nurses

British Medical Journal

"*Anyone Can Intubate* will give a good grounding lin intubation to anaesthetists starting training and to junior casualty officers as well as the the two groups mentioned above [nurses, ambulancemen]..." "I recommend the book as an adjunct to the practical training of anaesthetists and for those others who may from time to time be required to perform emergency intubation." — **David G. Price**

Anesthesia and Anaalgesia

"This unpretentious little book provides an excellent overview for the neophyte and can be read in an evening." — **Joanne C. Hudson, MD**

Journal of Royal Army Medical Corps

"Anyone who follows the precepts laid down here will be safe to be let loose on patients. I would recommend this book to all Anaesthetic departments with trainees and I shall be chaining up my personal copy!." — **H B Hannah**

Anyone Can Intubate

4th Edition

Christine E. Whitten, MD

Chief of Perioperative Services
Kaiser Permanente Hospital, San Diego, California

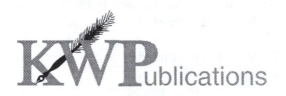

KWPublications

San Diego, California 92196

Ordering Information (see p. 239 for an order form)
Additional copies of this book may be purchased at your local bookstore specializing in professional or medical books or directly from the publisher at the address below. Remit $19.95 plus $3.50 for postage. California residents add sales tax.

For information concerning bulk purchases or course adoptions write or call:
K-W Publications
P.O. BOX 26455, San Diego, California 92196
1-800-450-2665 (8 a.m. - 5 p.m., Pacific Coast Time)

Copyright © 1989, 1990, 1994, 1997 by Christine E. Whitten, MD
Illustrations Copyrighted © 1989, 1990, 1994, 1997 by Christine E. Whitten, MD

All rights reserved. No part of this book shall be reproduced, stored in a retrieval system, or transmitted by any means, electronic, mechanical, photocopying, recording, or otherwise, without written permission from the publisher. This book is intended for the use of practicing medical professionals or students of those professions studying under the supervision of a trained medical instructor. It is not intended for use by lay people outside the profession.

Design by Mike Kelly, K-W Publications, San Diego, CA 92196

Library of Congress Catalog Card Number: 94-075815

Softcover: ISBN 0-929894-18-9

Printing History: 1st ed. published January 1989, 2d ed. January 1990, 3rd ed. April 1994, 4th ed. January 1997.

Printed in the United States of America
10 9 8 7 6 5 4 3

CONTENTS

Acknowledgements 9
Introduction 10

Chapter 1:   Anatomy 12
Single Cartilages 12
Paired Cartilages 16
Tying It All Together — Membranes and Muscles 16
Anatomy of the Lower Airway 19

Chapter 2:   Pulmonary Physiology and Assessing Respiration 25
Some Definitions 25
Control of Respiration 26
Oxygenation and Oxygen Delivery 29
Lung Volumes 33
Ventilation vs. Blood Flow: V/Q Mismatch 37
Intubation Criteria 38

Chapter 3:   Establishing an Airway 42
Recognizing Airway Obstruction 42
Use of the Nasal Airway 47
Use of the Oral Airway 48
Ventilating With a Bag and a Mask 50

Chapter 4:   Preintubation Evaluation
— Predicting the Difficult Airway 60
Medical History 60
Physical Signs 60

Chapter 5:   Equipment 68
Checking Your Laryngoscope 69
Checking Your Endotracheal Tube 70
Placing Your Stylet 71
Final Details 72
What To Do When You Don't Have Optimal
    Equipment 73

Chapter 6:   **Oral Intubation of the Adult 74**
The Dummy vs. the Real Thing 74
Intubating the Adult 75
Securing the Tube 85
Straight vs. Curved Blades 86

Chapter 7:   **Common Errors and How To Avoid Them 93**
Positioning Errors 93
Left-handed Intubation 94
Problems with Techniques 95

Chapter 8:   **Tests for Tube Placement 99**
Seven Steps for Correct Tube Placement 99
Esophageal Intubations 100
Mainstem Intubation 101
Tube Is Too Shallow 102

Chapter 9:   **Ventilating and Intubating the Child 104**
Children Are Not Small Adults 104
Equipment for Pediatric Intubation 109
Intubating the Infant 110
Intubating the Child 112

Chapter 10:   **Nasal Intubation Techniques 113**
Indications and Contraindications 113
Anatomy 114
Techniques 114

Chapter 11:   **Studies in Difficult Intubations:**
     Tricks of the Trade 125
    Cardiac Arrest 125
    Obesity 129
    Through the Veil: Partial Plates and Cleft Palates 131
    Edentulous 132
    Receding Chins 132
    Overbites 133
    Poor Neck Mobility 133
    Fixed Airway Obstruction 136
    Blood in the Oropharynx 140
    The Use of Cricoid Pressure 140
    A Difficult Intubation Algorithm 141

Chapter 12:   **Airway Management of Trauma 144**
    Airway Evaluation 144
    Airway Management 146
    Adjuncts to Intubation 153
    Special Considerations 154
    Stress and the Caregiver 162

Chapter 13:   **Specialized Ventilation Techniques 164**
    Esophageal Obturator Airway 164
    Laryngeal Mask Airway 166
    Esophageal-Tracheal Combitube 177
    Needle Cricothyroidotomy and Jet Ventilation 177
    Surgical Cricothyroidotomy 181

Chapter 14:   **Specialized Intubating Equipment 184**
Safeguarding Patient Safety 184
Flexible Guides 185
Manipulating Endotracheal Tubes, Blades,
    and Handles 188
Flexible Fiberoptic Bronchoscopes 194
Retrograde Wires 200
Combining Anterograde Fiberoptic
    Bronchoscopy with a Retrograde Wire 201
The Laryngeal Mask Airway as a Guide 203
Rigid Bronchoscopy 203

Chapter 15:   **Awake Intubation 204**
Risks of Using Sedation 204
Factors Influencing Drug Effect 206
Evaluating the Effect of Sedation 206
Local Anesthesia of the Oropharynx 207

Chapter 16:   **Induction Agents and Muscle Relaxants 211**
Preparing the Patient 212
Indications for Rapid Sequence Induction of
    Anesthesia 212
Relative Contraindications 213
Use of Induction Agents 214
Pharmacology of Muscle Relaxants 216
Reversal of Muscle Relaxation 220

Chapter 17:   **Extubating and Exchanging Endotracheal Tubes 222**
Extubation 222
Changing an Endotracheal Tube 226

Chapter 18:   **Complications 229**
Complications Occurring During the Intubation 229
Complications Occurring While Intubated 231
Complications Following Extubation 233

Index 235
About the Author 238
Order Form 239

To my parents
Ward and Bettye Whitten
— for all the years of
encouragement and belief.

Acknowledgements

No book is ever written alone. I wish to express my deep appreciation
for all the help and constructive criticism. I especially wish to thank
Doctors James Crawford, Susan Dickerson, Michael Dickerson,
Clyde Jones, Suzanne Quenneville, Diane Rand, and Anne Wong for
their technical reviews and support. Special thanks to my husband
Michael D. Kelly whose inspiration and expert knowledge in editing,
design, and computers made this book possible.

Correspondence to the author

Please address correspondence to Dr. Christine E. Whitten
c/o KW Publications, P.O. Box 26455, San Diego, CA 92196.

Manuscripts Requested

KW Publications is accepting manuscripts for review for subjects in
the medical field. Please write with your proposals to:
P.O. Box 26455, San Diego, CA 92196.

INTRODUCTION

To intubate means to place an endotracheal tube into the trachea. It's a life-saving skill. Hospitals today expect most doctors, nurses, medical students, nursing students, paramedics, and respiratory technicians to be able to ventilate and intubate any patient.

I've trained many people to intubate in my career as an anesthesiologist. The literature available to learn the basic technique of intubation is very limited. Most texts discuss intubation with the expert in mind. They give a short description of technique accompanied by one or two pictures of the head in cross-section. They lack detailed instruction because intubation has been a skill passed from mentor to student by long apprenticeship. Today's increasing emphasis on teaching large numbers of students the technique during short training sessions requires a different type of textbook. My book is designed to fill that need.

Anyone Can Intubate starts with the essential airway anatomy.

Chapter 2 then gives a brief review of respiratory physiology. This chapter is not essential to learning how to intubate or ventilate a patient. However, some understanding of physiology is very helpful in assessing the need for intubation as well as in evaluating how well you are ventilating a patient. Often when you know why you are doing something a certain may it makes it easier to learn how to do it.

Chapter 3 then discusses techniques in ventilating the patient with a bag and mask apparatus and offers tips for treating airway obstruction. Both skills are just as important as intubation itself.

With words and pictures you'll then learn how to manipulate airway anatomy in order to intubate. You'll find step-by-step instruction on how to place your hands, move the head, and handle the instruments in a safe and effective manner. You'll learn why each move is important and what it accomplishes. This makes the technique easier to master and it puts you in control. Heavy reliance on illustrations makes visualizing the steps of intubation easier.

Anyone Can Intubate won't replace hands-on practice with a mannequin. However, it *will* tell you how intubating the mannequin differs from the real patient, something often skipped in short courses. This difference often startles and hinders the beginning intubator the first time he or she makes the transition to a patient.

In addition to routine adult oral and nasal intubation we'll also look at pediatric intubation. Since children's anatomy is different, intubating pediatric patients is different.

You'll also learn:

- how to alter your technique when faced with a challenging or difficult intubation,
- steps to take if you cannot intubate the patient,
- strategies for managing the airway during cardiac arrests and other emergencies,

The text has been extensively revised to make it more useful for the physician in the emergency room as well as the paramedic in the field. Chapters have been added or revised to detail:

- strategies for managing the traumatized airway;
- the indications, contraindications, and techniques for emergency intubation under general anesthesia;
- the use of specialized equipment such as the fiberoptic laryngoscope, laryngeal mask airway, esophageal obturator airway, and the esophageal-tracheal combitube;
- criteria for assessing the patient's readiness for extubation;
- techniques for exchanging endotracheal tubes;
- strategies for the safe use of sedation;
- techniques for performing nerve blocks of the airway.

Anyone Can Intubate gives you a visual picture of intubation. As you proceed through the book, picture yourself performing the steps. Understand why moving the patient's head in a certain way, or changing the angle of your laryngoscope blade alters your view. See the anatomy in your mind's eye. Practice intubation at every available opportunity. Rereading this text after such practice will improve your comprehension and retention.

While intubation is a skill that requires practice to master, *anyone* can intubate.

1 ANATOMY

To intubate, you have to manipulate the anatomy to see the best view of the larynx. This is very difficult to do if you don't know how all the structures tie together. Knowledge of normal anatomy lets you identify the landmarks — even when faced with abnormal anatomy.

When you intubate, you place the endotracheal tube between the vocal cords and through a complex structure known as the **larynx**. The larynx is nothing more than a sophisticated valve with a variety of functions. We breathe through our larynx. It protects our airway from **aspiration**, the inhalation of foreign material. Its regulation of lung pressures generates the force required to cough. The larynx vibrates the air column to alter pitch and loudness when we speak. It can do these things because of its unique structure.

To feel your own larynx, place your hand on the front of your neck. Identify the firm, roughly cylindrical shape in the midline. Your Adam's apple is part of your larynx (Fig. 1-1, 1-2).

The larynx sits on top of the trachea opposite the fourth, fifth, and sixth cervical vertebrae in the adult. It's a boxlike structure composed of nine cartilages connected by ligaments and moved by nine muscles (Fig. 1-3, 1-4). Far from a static structure, these three single and three paired cartilages pivot and swing in relationship to each other. The connections between the cartilages are true joints with a built-in range of motion. Movement of the surrounding tissues shifts the cartilages as well.

Single Cartilages

The single cartilages form the basic structure of the larynx and provide us with our major external landmarks.

The **cricoid ring** is signet shaped, with the broad aspect posterior. It sits on

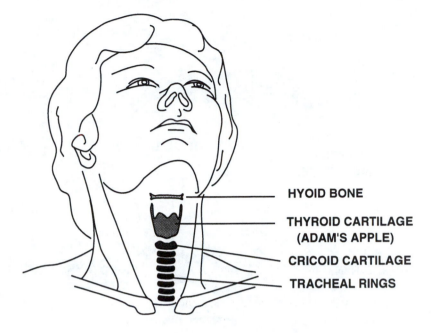

Fig. 1-1. The larynx from the front.

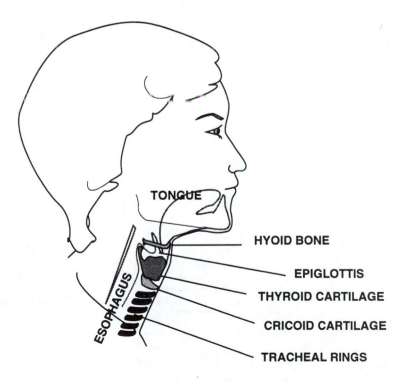

Fig. 1-2. Profile of the larynx.

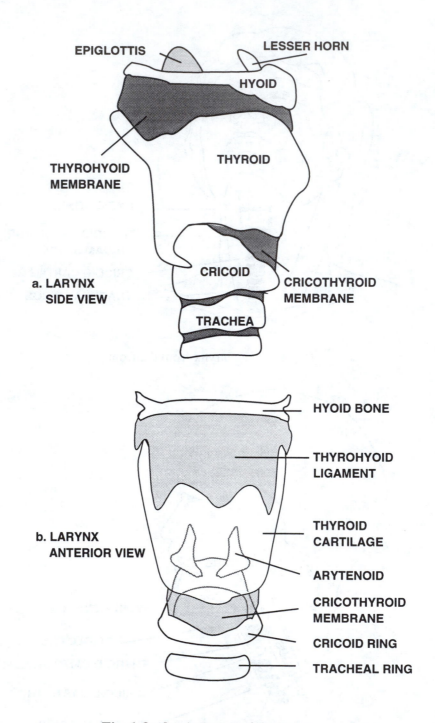

EPIGLOTTIS

LESSER HORN

HYOID

THYROHYOID
MEMBRANE

THYROID

a. LARYNX
SIDE VIEW

CRICOID

CRICOTHYROID
MEMBRANE

TRACHEA

HYOID BONE

THYROHYOID
LIGAMENT

b. LARYNX
ANTERIOR VIEW

THYROID
CARTILAGE

ARYTENOID

CRICOTHYROID
MEMBRANE

CRICOID RING

TRACHEAL RING

Fig. 1-3a, b. Anatomy of the larynx.

top of the first tracheal ring. To easily feel this cartilage, place your fingers on the trachea in the sternal notch and slide them upward. You'll feel a firm, incompressible, ring shaped structure about three to four fingers breadth above the notch. This nondistensible ring is the smallest diameter in the child's airway. Two cricothyroid joints connect the ring anteriorly to the thyroid cartilage, allowing the two to move both independently and as a unit.

The **thyroid cartilage** consists of two quadrangular plates fused anteriorly in

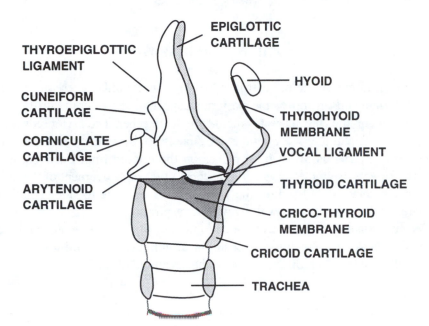

a. LARYNX, CROSS SECTION — SIDE VIEW

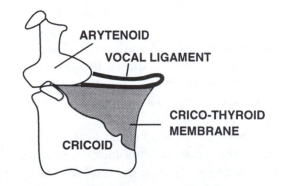

b. CRICO/ARYTENOID COMPLEX — SIDE VIEW

Fig. 1-4a, b. Cross-section of the larynx.

the midline. You also know this cartilage as the Adam's apple. Feel this cartilage as a firm projection in the midline of the neck just superior to the cricoid ring. There is a notch on its top edge.

The **epiglottis** is a curved, leaf shaped structure whose upper, rounded edge projects into the pharynx. The stalk of the leaf connects anteriorly to the inside of the thyroid lamina at its midpoint. It also connects to the hyoid bone and to the base of the tongue. You can't feel the epiglottis externally, but it's a major visual landmark in the pharynx when you intubate.

Paired Cartilages

The most important paired cartilages are the **arytenoids**. These are irregular pyramids mounted on top of the posterior aspect of the cricoid cartilage. The signet flange on the ring separates them from each other. The arytenoids are important visual landmarks for intubation. You must be able to recognize their shape. The arytenoids pivot in all planes on the cricoid ring. Each vocal cord projects forward from the sharp anterior vocal process. Movement of the arytenoids tenses, relaxes, and swings the vocal cords from side to side. This lets us phonate, breath, cough, and swallow without aspirating.

The cone shaped **corniculates** attach to the apex of the arytenoids and the elongated **cuneiforms** attach to the posterior arytenoids. They're important to us only because they add bulk and shape to the arytenoid outline.

Tying It All Together: Membranes and Muscles

Several ligaments and two membranes connect the laryngeal cartilages. The most important membrane is the **cricoid membrane**, which runs from the arytenoids to the thyroid cartilage. The upper free edge of this membrane is the vocal cord.

Normally, the cords are pale and pearly white. Their attachment to the cricoid ring both directly and indirectly explains the success of cricoid pressure. As you'll see, we use downward pressure on the cricoid ring to help bring the vocal cords into view when they are hidden behind the tongue. Pushing on the cricoid pushes the cords.

Structurally, the anterior two thirds is membranous and the posterior one third is cartilaginous. The cartilaginous skeleton allows the vocal cords to close the larynx more effectively if the need arises. It may prevent you from placing an endotracheal tube between closed cords. Forcing a tube through the cords with excessive pressure can actually dislocate an arytenoid and cause permanent hoarseness.

A second membrane, the **quadrangular membrane**, runs anteriorly from the lateral border of the arytenoids. The upper edge forms the aryepiglottic fold. The lower edge forms the vestibular fold or false vocal cord. The false cords thus lie above the true vocal cords and help close the glottis.

The entire larynx falls on inspiration and rises on expiration. It also rises on coughing, straining, and swallowing. This makes sense. A lower larynx opens the airway while a higher one places the epiglottis and the tongue in better position to close it. Place your hand on your larynx and you can feel the movements.

When at rest, the vocal cords lie partially separated, or abducted. During forceful inspiration or hyperventilation, the cords open widely, producing a lozenge shaped opening (Fig. 1-5). This minimizes resistance to breathing. Hyper–ventilation also makes it easier for us to pass an endotracheal tube in an awake patient.

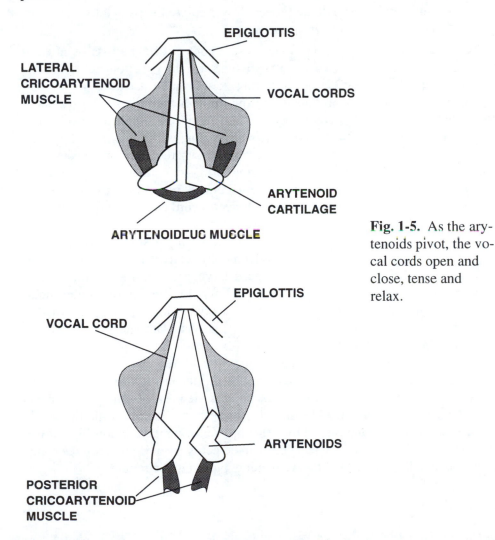

Fig. 1-5. As the arytenoids pivot, the vocal cords open and close, tense and relax.

To produce a high pitched voice, or in response to tracheobronchial irritation, the interarytenoid muscles pinch the cords together, or adduct them.

Injury to the recurrent laryngeal nerve produces vocal cord paralysis on the affected side. A paralyzed cord lies halfway between fully closed and fully open, the cadaveric position. The recurrent laryngeal nerve carries fibers which both separate and approximate the cords. It's easier to damage the more superficial separating fibers. Surgery or trauma sometimes bruises or cuts these fibers. Airway obstruction can occur if the vocal cord dysfunction occurs on both sides because the undamaged approximating fibers pull the cords together.

Closure of the larynx occurs by three mechanisms:

1. closure of the vocal cords

2. closure of the false cords

3. mounding of the paraglottic tissues (lower epiglottis, paraglottic fat, base of tongue) by elevation of the larynx.

The larynx depends so strongly on muscle control that the loss of muscle tone can cause airway obstruction. Soft tissue, including the tongue, falls into the airway and can block the opening. Muscle relaxation narrows the gap between the cords but does not alter gas flow through the larynx. The resultant Bernoulli effect sucks the cords together and produces a high pitched, noisy sound with respiration. This sound, known as **stridor**, is characteristic of airway obstruction. Obstruction can occur regardless of whether loss of muscle tone comes from unconsciousness, muscle relaxant drugs, or cardiac arrest.

By contrast, light anesthesia, excessive secretions, or aspiration stimulate the airway and activate the defense reflexes. Forceful cord closure and elevation of the larynx seal the airway. **Laryngospasm**, or spasmotic closure of the vocal cords, is the most severe form of airway closure. Airway obstruction from laryngospasm can totally prevent ventilation. It can physically prevent the passage of an endotracheal tube. You have experienced laryngospasm when you accidentally tried to aspirate water or a pea at dinner. Laryngospasm produced the choking sensation and the loud, stridorous noises you made when you finally succeeded in taking a breath. Carried to extreme your laryngeal protective reflexes prevent air exchange.

Let's turn to the actual appearance of the larynx. Although covered by mucous membrane, you can still see the basic, underlying skeletal shapes. Memorize the view from the top. Look for this view every time you intubate (Fig. 1-6). Try to picture how the underlying skeleton will move when you pull or push on the membrane draped over the top. Knowing the relationships of the structures will let you find the gap between the cords, even if you only see some of the landmarks. Understanding the anatomy puts you in control.

Anatomy of the Lower Airway

Knowledge of the lower airway and the dynamics of breathing are important to know when assessing a patient's respiration and when ventilating him.

Trachea and Lung

The trachea is about 10-12 cm long in the average adult. It extends from the cricoid cartilage down to the 6th cervical vertebrae where it splits into a right

FRONT OF THE PATIENT

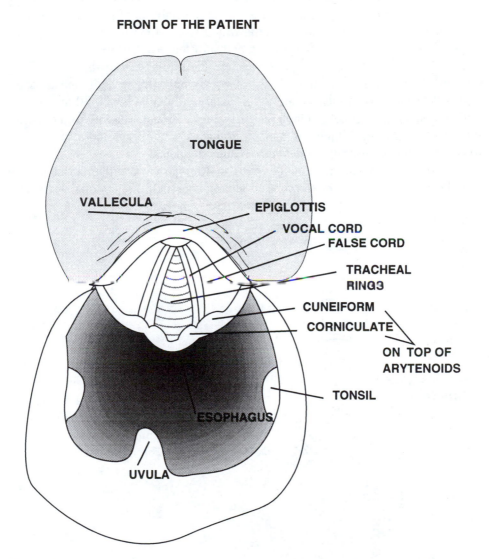

Fig. 1-6. Larynx viewed from the top. Front of the patient is at top of the page.

and left mainstem bronchus. The right mainstem bronchus comes off the trachea at a more vertical angle and is shorter. As a result, aspirated material or endotracheal tubes which are inserted too far tend to go down the right rather than the left side (Fig. 1-7).

The diameter of the trachea in an infant is 3 mm and grows about 1 mm a year until the adult diameter of about 15 mm is reached. Symptomatic airway obstruction at rest due to narrowing of the trachea or larynx usually does not occur until 70-80% of the diameter is lost. At this point, respirations sound harsh and "creaking" — due to air turbulence, a noise called stridor. Stridor is an indication of significant airway obstruction and needs to be managed aggressively.

The mucous membrane consists of 2 sets of specialized cells: one producing mucous and the other covered with cilia which sweep the mucous and any collected particulate matter up the trachea and into the oropharynx where they're swallowed. This process, plus coughing, removes debris from the lungs. The cilia are very sensitive to the effects of breathing cold, dry air and also to smoke. The smoke from one cigarette can paralyze the cilia for 20-30 minutes.

The 2 mainstem bronchi branch into the smaller bronchi leading to the major lobes of the lung. Each lung has 3 major divisions: an upper, middle, and lower lobe. Each lobe in turn subdivides into smaller segments.

The bronchi branch into smaller and smaller airways called bronchioles. Finally, off the smallest, or terminal bronchioles branch the alveolar ducts and

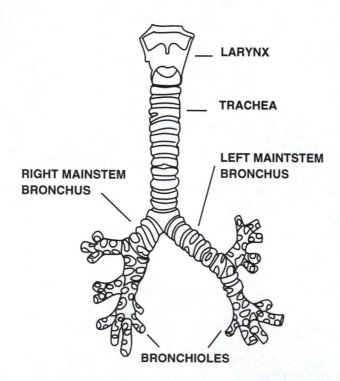

LARYNX

TRACHEA

LEFT MAINTSTEM BRONCHUS

RIGHT MAINSTEM BRONCHUS

BRONCHIOLES

Fig. 1-7. Tracheal Tree. The trachea divides into 2 mainstem bronchi and then into smaller divisions called bronchioles.

the alveoli. Alveoli are the microscopic air sacs where all of the air exchange takes place. There are 200-600 million alveoli in the normal lung having a total alveolar surface area of 40-100 square meters (Fig. 1-8). A cluster of alveoli on a terminal bronchiole along with their capillaries is called an **acinus**.

Each alveolus looks like a tiny balloon. Its 0.02 micron thick wall, which is the barrier to diffusion of oxygen and carbon dioxide, consists of the alveolar cell wall and its basement membrane separated from the capillary bed by loose connective tissue. Special cells inside the alveolus produce surfactant, a detergent-like substance that decreases the surface tension pulling the balloon closed. Decreased tension allows the alveoli to inflate more easily and with less pressure. Without surfactant, the alveoli would collapse.

The lung structure is fairly spongy. Once expanded from an inhalation, it passively and effortlessly returns to its resting state due to its elasticity. Expelling all of the air from the lungs in forced exhalation requires effort.

Oxygen passively diffuses through this wall into the capillaries where it is carried back via the pulmonary veins to the left side of the heart and distributed

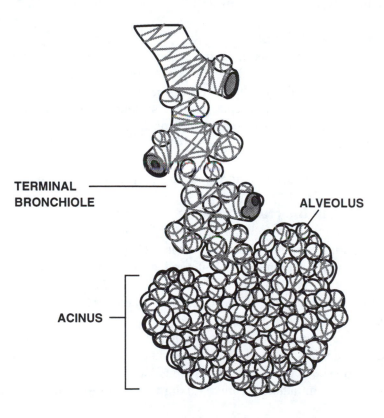

TERMINAL BRONCHIOLE

ALVEOLUS

ACINUS

Fig. 1-8. Alveoli. A cluster of alveoli on a terminal bronchiole is called an acinus. The capillary newwork is shown in gray.

to the rest of the body. Carbon dioxide passively leaves the capillaries to enter the alveoli, where it is then exhaled from the body.

For this system to function the alveoli must have free access to the inspired gas. Blockage of the bronchi or alveolar ducts prevents new oxygen from entering the alveoli and prevents carbon dioxide from leaving. This can occur with mucous plugging or foreign body aspiration.

Pneumonia is inflammation of the lungs produced by infection or chemical exposure. The alveoli fill with fluid, white cells, and debris, preventing gas exchange.

In emphysema, the lung is damaged, causing breakdown of alveolar walls. This produces enlarged alveoli which are present in decreasing numbers. The greatly decreased surface area for exchanging oxygen produces hypoxemia. The lungs begin to stay hyper-inflated all the time since the loss of alveoli causes the loss of lung elasticity. The lung does not passively collapse with exhalation. The diaphragm is pushed downward, becoming more flattened. With this relative mechanical disadvantage, the patient must work harder to take a breath, increasing the work of breathing. Carbon dioxide diffuses so freely that rarely is its passage impaired due to lung damage.

Pulmonary Blood Supply

The lungs have two sets of arteries. The right and left pulmonary arteries spring from the right ventricular outflow tract to bring venous blood from the right side of the heart to the lungs. Here it is oxygenated in the capillary beds surrounding the alveoli. A second arterial system called bronchiolar arteries brings oxygenated blood from the left side of the heart to the lung tissue, particularly the bronchioles.

Distribution of the blood in the lungs is controlled by two factors, pulmonary artery pressure compared to intra-pulmonary air pressure and gravity.

Diaphragm and Intercostal Muscles

The diaphragms are two large dome-shaped sheets of muscle separating the thoracic cavities from the abdominal cavity. They are supplied by the phrenic nerves, which originate in the neck at cervical nerve roots 3 through 5. The intercostal nerves supply the muscles between the ribs. Thus a cervical spinal cord injury at C6 will eliminate intercostal muscle function but allow breathing from maintained diaphragmatic function.

The diaphragm contracts with each inhalation, causing it to descend toward the abdomen and assume a more flattened shape. The intercostals also contract, pulling the ribs outward. Both these actions increase intrathoracic volume. The resulting drop in intrathoracic pressure. draws air into the lungs, which expand (Fig. 1-9).

During exhalation, the diaphragm and intercostals relax. The chest wall passively resumes its previous shape. The diaphragm returns to its resting dome shape and rises higher into the chest cavity. This decreases intrathoracic volume. Pressure inside the thorax rises and the patient passively exhales. Unless there is obstruction, exhalation is passive, requiring little energy.

This system is very efficient during normal spontaneous respiration. Things change during manual ventilation. During manual ventilation, enough positive pressure must be applied to an open airway to expand the lungs by actively filling the alveoli. The chest wall must be lifted and the diaphragms pushed downward, displacing the abdominal contents to do so. If the airway is not held open, the gas will often take the path of least resistance and enter the stomach, producing distension and increasing the risk of vomiting. A distended stomach then pushes on the diaphragm and ventilation becomes even more difficult.

Conditions which make ventilation difficult are:

- increased intra-abdominal pressure which limits descent of the diaphragm, such as obesity or pregnancy;

- increased intra-thoracic pressure, such as pneumothorax;

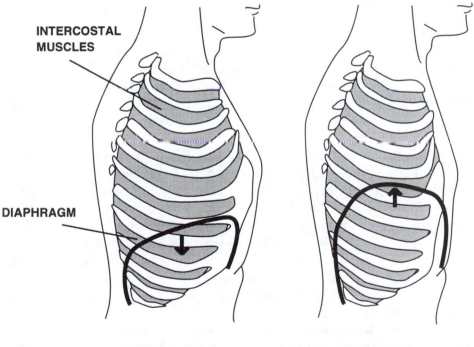

INSPIRATION   **EXPIRATION**

Fig. 1-9. Diaphragm. On inspiration the diaphragm and intercostal muscles contact, expanding the chest cavity. Air enters the lungs. On expiration the muscles relax, allowing passive exhalation.

- poor pulmonary compliance, such as pneumonia where alveoli are filled with fluid or asthma where the bronchioles are in spasm;
- upper airway obstruction;
- lower airway obstruction.

The basic techniques of how to open the airway and how to ventilate will be covered in Chapter 3.

Problems can also arise if the system is damaged. For example, if a pneumothorax is present, then expansion of the chest cavity no longer drops the intrathoracic pressure as much. If the pressure change is large enough the lung may only partially expand or may not expand at all. If the pressure rises over baseline in that hemi-thorax, the increased pressure can push the heart and other lung over, producing a tension pneumothorax. This is a life-threatening situation requiring decompression of the chest to allow ventilation.

Alternatively, if a diaphragm is paralyzed by phrenic nerve damage, then that diaphragm will, paradoxically, move with breathing. It will move upward during inspiration and downward during expiration. The patient's tidal volume decreases and his work of breathing increases. The patient with marginal respiratory reserve may need assistance.

Chest Wall

The ribs form three functional groupings. The first rib attaches rigidly to the sternum and serves to anchor the rib cage. It hardly moves during respiration. The 2nd through 7th ribs flexibly expand in two dimensions with each inhalation: anterior-posteriorly and laterally. The 8th through 12th ribs expand mostly laterally during inspiration, effectively increasing the intra-abdominal space for the organs pushed downward by the diaphragm.

The angulation and compliance of the ribs during the breathing cycle maximizes efficiency in the adult. Full contraction of the intercostals and the diaphragm allows for significant expansion of the chest cavity and produces a large breath. In the infant or small child, the ribs are less angled. To take a deep breath the infant's chest expands a little and the abdomen rises a lot as the diaphragm descends, pushing abdominal contents down and out of the way. Babies "belly breathe". Anything which interferes with descent of the diaphragm, such as a stomach distended with air, can seriously impair an infant's breathing. Decompression of the stomach should be considered in the infant or small child with respiratory distress.

The infant's chest wall is also more compliant. When the infant takes a breath against resistance, such as airway obstruction, the chest wall actually moves inward as the belly moves outward. The inward movement of the chest wall decreases the amount of air which enters. The baby must work harder to breathe and may tire if this effort goes on too long.

2 PULMONARY PHYSIOLOGY AND ASSESSING RESPIRATION

U nderstanding a bit about the physiology of respiration is not essential to learning the techniques of how to intubate or how to ventilate; but it will give you a better means of assessing the status of the patient. It will help you decide what you need to do to optimize the patient's ventilation and whether you need to intubate. To this end we'll look at :

- control of respiration;
- some simple chemistry of how the body handles carbon dioxide and maintains its acid/base balance;
- oxygenation and oxygen delivery;
- lung volumes and how they can change;
- gas distribution related to blood distribution or V/Q matching; and
- intubation criteria.

Some Definitions

Physiology is the study of how the body functions. To function optimally, the body's cells and organs must be surrounded by a specific environment, consisting of an optimal range of blood acidity (pH), arterial oxygen level (P_aO_2), arterial carbon dioxide level (P_aCO_2), and temperature, among other things. This optimal range can be disrupted by external factors such as exposure to cold without adequate clothing, breathing low oxygen gases, or starvation. The optimal range is more commonly disrupted by internal factors, such as infections, traumatic damage, and progressive disfunction caused by such things as aging and smoking.

When minor physiologic changes occur, the body compensates to continue to function. If the changes are too great or too prolonged then the body may ultimately decompensate.

The following sections will define new terms as they appear. In general, when you see a small subscript "a," as in P_aO_2, this refers to arterial blood values. A small subscript "v" refers to venous blood. A subscript capital "A" refers to alveolar, or intrapulmonary gas values.

Control of Respiration

Sensing Changes in CO_2 and pH

The respiratory "center" is found in the midbrain, comprised of sections of both the medulla and pons. This center determines the rate and depth of respirations based on feedback from chemical stimuli in the blood.

Respiration varies throughout the course of the day depending on the patient's need and on the feedback signals received by the brain. **Hypoventilation** means that not enough respiration is occurring to support oxygen demands and to eliminate the CO_2 being produced. **Hyperventilation** means there is increased pulmonary ventilation beyond that needed to maintain the blood gas levels within the normal range. The most important stimuli for respiration are the level of carbon dioxide, the acid/base balance, and the level of oxygen.

To start each normal respiration, a signal travels from the brain down the phrenic and intercostal nerves to cause a person to inhale. The respiratory rate will often change to try to counteract any changes in the tension of oxygen, carbon dioxide, and acid in the blood stream. The level of carbon dioxide in the arterial blood stream is called the P_aCO_2. The level of oxygen in the arterial blood is called the P_aO_2. The "P" refers to the partial pressure of the dissolved gas in the blood, measured in mmHg. The term **mmHg** refers to millimeters of mercury, the same units used for barometric pressure.

The most powerful stimulus tends to be the level of carbon dioxide, or P_aCO_2, in the bloodstream because of its effect on the pH. Small changes in P_aCO_2 cause significant changes in pH and thus in ventilatory drive.

The symbol **pH** is a measure of relative acidity. Neutral pH equals 7.0. When the concentration of hydrogen ions, or H^+, goes up, the pH goes down and the solution is said to be acidic. As H^+ goes down, the pH goes up, and the solution becomes more basic. The normal balance of acid to base in blood produces a pH of about 7.35 – 7.45. This pH must be maintained for optimal enzyme function in the cells. The normal blood concentration, or partial pressure, of carbon dioxide (CO_2) is 35 – 45 mmHg.

The changes in pH are brought about according to the chemical reaction:

$$CO_2 + H_2O \rightleftharpoons H_2CO_3 \rightleftharpoons H^+ + HCO_3^-$$

What this formula means is that carbon dioxide is highly reactive with water and when combined with water will form acetic acid (H_2CO_3). Acetic acid will then break up into positively and negatively charged ions in such a way as to keep the blood acid/base balance as neutral as possible. The bloodstream normally has a certain amount of the base bicarbonate (HCO_3^-) in solution which helps to buffer or neutralize any acids being produced.

As carbon dioxide levels rise above normal — a state called **hypercarbia** — the chemical reaction shifts to the right and produces more hydrogen ions (H^+). If there are more hydrogen ions in solution than bicarbonate ions (HCO_3^-), the solution becomes more acidic.

The blood will also become more acidic if the amount of HCO_3^- falls, such as from certain types of kidney dysfunction. Acidity will also rise if the amount of H^+ rises, such as from lactic acid production during shock or hypoxia.

Whatever the cause of rising acidity, the respiratory center will produce an increase in respiratory rate and depth to compensate. The resultant hyperventilation drops the level of CO_2 in the bloodstream, the chemical reaction shifts to the left, and the blood becomes less acid. Most of the time this compensation is beneficial.

The compensatory mechanism can sometimes be harmful. For example, when a patient hyperventilates, perhaps in response to anxiety or pain, the P_aCO_2 drops and the blood pH rises. A level of P_aCO_2 less than baseline is called **hypocarbia**. Hypocarbia causes vasoconstriction and decreases blood flow to the major organs, including the brain. If the P_aCO_2 is less than 20 mmHg, the brain will not have enough oxygen to function normally. Whenever an organ lacks enough oxygen it is said to be **ischemic**. Ischemia causes localized acidosis in the cerebral spinal fluid. This local acidosis can continue to promote the hyperventilation. A vicious cycle starts. Having a hyperventilating patient breathe into a paper bag allows him to rebreathe his own CO_2, raising his blood P_aCO_2 and thus breaking the cycle.

When you ventilate a patient who is likely to be acidotic, it's important to hyperventilate the patient slightly to try to compensate and bring the pH back toward normal. However, too much hyperventilation, as we just described, is not necessarily a good thing. Having blood gas results available to guide your assisted ventilation is optimal but not always available.

Other Conditions Effecting the Respiratory Center

Drugs and the status of the patient will effect the sensitivity of the respiratory center. Narcotics are one of the most common types of drugs effecting the center. They effectively raise the "set point," causing the center to accept a higher level of P_aCO_2 as normal. As a result, patients will decrease their respiratory rate and depth in a dose dependent fashion until the higher P_aCO_2 is reached. If the dose of narcotic is high enough, the patient will become apneic.

This relationship also means that if the patient is manually ventilated to a

$PaCO_2$ lower than her current "set-point" she will stop breathing. For example, if the patient's "set-point" says a P_aCO_2 of 50 mmHg is normal because of narcotic administration, and the P_aCO_2 is now 40 mmHg, the patient may not breathe. It's very common to see this phenomenon in anesthetized patients. To get the patient to start breathing, the anesthesia provider gradually decreases the rate and depth of ventilation to allow the P_aCO_2 to rise, while at the same time maintaining adequate oxygenation. As soon as the P_aCO_2 goes above the patient's "set-point," she will begin to breathe. You will also commonly see this occur when trying to wean a patient from the ventilator.

Continuously high levels of CO_2 above 70 mmHg will desensitize the respiratory center to CO_2. The primary driving force to breathe then becomes the level of oxygen or P_aO_2, which is a weaker stimulus than hypercarbia. When the level of oxygen drops too low for normal body function, the patient is said to be **hypoxic**. A patient who depends on the low level of oxygen in her bloodstream to stimulate her to breathe is said to be dependent on her **hypoxic drive**, and is diagnosed as a **CO_2 retainer**. An example of this type of patient is one with chronically high CO_2 due to end stage emphysema. When you administer a high concentration of oxygen to this type of patient you may take away her drive to breathe and cause her to hypoventilate or to stop breathing. More on the acute management of the CO_2 retainer later in this chapter.

Sepsis, probably through the effect of endotoxin on the respiratory center, is a very powerful stimulus to increase respiratory rate and depth. Other conditions increasing ventilation are pulmonary embolus, shock, fear, fever, and pain. Anything which tends to turn on the sympathetic nervous system tends to increase respiratory rate.

There is always a balance in each patient between the stimuli to increase and to decrease the respiratory drive. Bear this in mind as you treat your patient. An excellent example is the exhausted, hypoxemic patient with respiratory distress who is also afraid, in pain, and facing an awake intubation. This patient has powerful negative and positive drives to breathe. A small dose of narcotic and sedative to relieve her anxiety may be enough to tip the balance and produce apnea. Monitor such patients carefully.

Hypoventilation Causes Hypoxemia

Hypoventilation is a common cause of too little oxygen in the blood when the patient is breathing room air because the CO_2 takes up a significant amount of the space in the alveoli available for oxygen. The concentration of oxygen in the alveoli can be calculated using the Alveolar Gas Equation:

$$PAO_2 = FiO_2 (P_B - P_{H_2O}) - P_ACO_2 / R$$

Where:

PAO_2 = partial pressure of oxygen in the alveoli

FiO2 = concentration of inspired oxygen

PB = the barometric pressure where the patient is breathing

PH20 = the partial pressure of water in the air (usually 47 mmHg)

PACO2 = alveolar carbon dioxide tension

R = respiratory quotient, a constant usually assumed to be 0.8

Let's say that our patient at sea level breathing room air has a P_ACO_2 of 80 mmHg, or twice normal. Then the PAO2 calculates out to be:

$$PAO_2 = .21 (760 - 47) - 80/0.8 = 49 \text{ mmHg}$$

This is quite hypoxic, especially since the alveolar P_AO_2 is always a little higher than the arterial P_aO_2. Now let's put this patient on 50% oxygen and see what happens:

$$P_AO_2 = .5 (760 - 47) - 80/0.8 = 256 \text{ mmHg}$$

Putting the patient on oxygen will buy you time for treatment. If this is a quickly reversible process, such as a narcotic overdose, you may not need to intubate. However, if this is not quickly reversible, then oxygen buys you time to prepare your equipment for manual ventilation or intubation.

Let's go back to our CO_2 retaining emphysema patient relying on her hypoxic drive, which by the way, is only a very small minority of patients with emphysema. This patient was placed on 50% oxygen upon arrival to the hospital and the first blood gas showed her P_aO_2 was 45 and her P_aCO_2 was 85. The wrong thing to do would be to take all the oxygen off this patient in order to stimulate her breathing. As we saw in our example above, we'd expect the P_AO_2 to abruptly drop to 49 with this change. A better way would be to wean the oxygen back slowly. Intubation might be needed.

Sensing Changes in Oxygen

The sensors detecting the oxygen tension in the arterial blood, or P_aO_2, are located in the carotid bodies at the bifurcation of the carotid artery. Unlike the CO_2 sensors, the carotid bodies never get used to lower oxygen levels and will continue to detect it even in patients with chronic hypoxia. In contrast, the respiratory center does not respond to minor changes in oxygen. It often doesn't react to a decrease in FiO_2, until it falls to about 15% at sea level.

Oxygenation and Oxygen Delivery

Pulmonary Oxygenation

The FiO_2 for room air is 21%. Sick and injured patients often require more oxygen than this. Air exhaled from a person at rest typically contains $16 - 17\%$ oxygen. One of the main disadvantages of mouth to mouth ventilation is that unless the provider breathes enriched oxygen herself, the patient will receive no more than 17% oxygen, and probably less.

The normal P_aO_2 varies with age and can be estimated by the formula:

$$PaO_2 = 102 - 0.33 \text{ (age in years) mmHg}$$

The normal PaO_2 is also roughly equal to 5 times the FiO_2. Thus a patient breathing 40% FiO_2 will have a P_aO_2 of about 200 mmHg. A patient breathing room air, or 21% FiO_2, will have a P_aO_2 of 100 mmHg. Knowing this relationship lets you know whether the patient is relatively hypoxemic or not relative to the inspired FiO_2.

Hypoxemia refers to a subnormal concentration of oxygen in the blood. **Hypoxia** refers to an insufficient amount of oxygen in the tissues. The distinction is important. A patient breathing an FiO_2 of 50% oxygen who has a P_aO_2 of 100 is relatively hypoxemic — his P_aO_2 should be about 250 with that FiO_2. But he's not hypoxic, since a P_aO_2 of 100 provides a normal amount of oxygen to his tissues. On the other hand, a patient with a P_aO_2 of 50 is both hypoxic and hypoxemic.

Another important distinction to master is the difference between P_aO_2 and oxygen saturation. The P_aO_2, as we have seen, is the level of oxygen in the arterial blood in mmHg. **Oxygen saturation** (often abbreviated O_2 sat) is the percent of Hgb in the blood which is carrying oxygen. People sometimes confuse the two. The relationship appears in the Oxygen-Hemoglobin Dissociation Curve shown in Fig. 2-1. Since a normal P_aO_2 is between 90-100 mmHg, they may think that an O_2 sat of 90 is normal as well. This is very wrong.

An O_2 sat of 90% corresponds to a P_aO_2 of 60 mmHg. This is the minimum oxygen saturation which provides enough oxygen to resting tissues. Once the O_2 sat falls below 90%, the P_aO_2 drops precipitously into the dangerously hypoxic range.

When giving supplemental oxygen, try to keep the FiO_2 as low as possible while still providing adequate oxygenation. Over time, high levels of oxygen can be toxic to the lungs. Breathing $80 - 100\%$ oxygen for more than 24 hours can cause pulmonary congestion and edema. An FiO_2 less than $40 - 50\%$ even for prolonged periods appears to be safe. The concern for oxygen toxicity should never interfere with the acute stabilization of the patient.

Hypoxemia is not by itself an indication for intubation. It may not even be abnormal. For example, a healthy person living in Salt Lake City at altitude will have an O_2 sat of about 93% and a PaO_2 of about 65 mmHg. Although the FiO_2 is the same 21% in Salt Lake, the atmospheric pressure is less and therefore the number of molecules of oxygen floating in the air is less. He is hypoxemic, but normal. He compensates by having a higher red blood cell count and Hgb and a

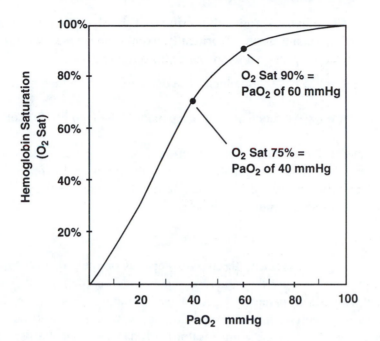

Fig. 2-1. Oxygen Hemoglobin Dissociation Curve showing the % of oxygen binding to hemoglobin (Hgb) for each PaO_2. Note how quickly hemoglobin loses oxygen below an O_2 sat of 90%.

tendency to hyperventilate a bit compared to sea level. By comparison, this means that our patient in Salt Lake has far less reserve than one at sea level and if injured may require more aggressive oxygen support.

Oxygen Content

Blood passing through the pulmonary capillaries picks up oxygen in 2 forms: bound to hemoglobin and dissolved in the serum. The vaste majority is bound to hemoglobin (Hgb). You can calculate the amount of oxygen content in the blood with the following formula.

O_2 content (cc/100 ml blood) = $O2$ bound to Hgb + O_2 dissolved

O_2 content = (Hgb x % sat x 1.39) + (PaO_2 x 0.003)

A patient with a normal PaO_2 of 100 has only 0.3 cc of oxygen dissolved in 100 ml of serum.

By contrast, if the Hgb is 12 and the O_2 sat is 100, then the amount of oxygen bound to Hgb will be:

O_2 bound to Hgb = 12 x 1.39 x 100/100 = 16.68 cc/100 ml blood

The total oxygen content in our example is 16.68 + 0.3 = 16.98 cc. The concentration of Hgb in the blood is thus critical. If the Hgb in a trauma patient is 5, then the oxygen content will fall critically, even if the PaO_2 stays 100:

O_2 content = (5 x 1.39 x 100/100) + (100 x 0.003)

O_2 content = 7.25 cc/100 ml blood or a decrease of more than half.

This is the same oxygen content as if our patient had a Hgb of 12 , but an O_2 sat of 43%.

As you can see, the development of anemia, from any cause, places the patient at risk for poor tissue oxygenation, even if the lungs are performing well and the Hgb is fully saturated. This is one reason why trauma patients need aggressive respiratory monitoring and support.

Oxygen Delivery

Providing adequate oxygen to the tissues depends on the amount of oxygen bound to Hgb in the blood and the cardiac output. Normal ventilation and blood oxygen content won't do the patient any good if cardiac output is poor. Thus, manual ventilation without chest compressions in a cardiac arrest victim is useless.

However, one of the prime compensatory mechanisms that the patient has when facing low blood oxygen content is a higher cardiac output. Patients develop tachycardia and increased stroke volume. This increased cardiac output moves more Hgb carrying red blood cells through the lungs to pick up oxygen and through the tissues to deliver it. A patient with low oxygen content for any reason won't tolerate bradycardia and low cardiac output, which will worsen hypoxemia. The combination of low oxygen content and decreased cardiac output can be rapidly fatal and you must guard against it.

Patients living at high altitude or those with chronic respiratory failure will develop high red blood cell counts to increase the amount of available Hgb to compensate. These patients depend on their higher levels of Hgb to function and will develop organ ischemia more readily if their Hgb is allowed to drop significantly — even if it drops to what would be a normal value in the average young adult. Thus, the question of what represents an acceptable Hgb really depends on the patient's clinical status and geographic location. The decision of when to transfuse will thus vary from patient to patient.

Another compensatory mechanism is how easily the hemoglobin releases or dissociates from the oxygen molecules. Conditions which cause Hgb to release oxygen more easily are fever, blood acidity, and an increased P_aCO_2 — conditions which are usually associated with increased oxygen requirements. Chronic hypoxia will cause the blood cell to produce more of the enzyme 2-3 DPG, which also allows the Hgb to give up oxygen even more readily. When Hgb releases oxygen more easily, the oxygen-hemoglobin dissociation curve shown in Fig. 2-1 shifts to the right.

Hypothermia, low P_aCO_2, and a higher pH cause the curve to shift to the left, meaning that Hgb holds on to oxygen more strongly. This is a potentially harmful disadvantage to an hypoxic patient. Avoid or treat these conditions aggressively when the patient is hypoxemic.

Lung Volumes

In addition to anatomical divisions into lobes and segments, the lungs are also divided into functional regions. These functional regions are called volumes and capacities. The lung volumes are defined as follows:

Tidal Volume (TV): the amount of air moved into and out of the lung during normal quiet breathing.

Inspiratory Reserve Volume (IRV): the maximum amount of air that can be inhaled after a normal inhalation

Expiratory Reserve Volume (ERV): the maxiumum amount of air which can be exhaled after a normal exhalation.

Reserve Volume (RV): the amount of air remaining in the lungs after exhaling as much as possible. The lungs never completely deflate.

Lung capacities are combinations of volumes.

Total Lung Capacity (TLC): the total volume of the lungs when they are maximally inflated. TLC = IRV + TV + ERV + RV

Forced Vital Capacity (FVC): the volume of air that a patient can exhale after a maximal inhaltion. FVC= IRV + ERV + TV

Functional Residual Capacity (FRC): the amount of air left in the lung after a normal exhalation. FRC = ERV + RV

Inspiratory Capacity (IC): theamount of air that can be inhaled after a normal exhalation. IC = TV + IRV

Vital Capacity (VC): the total lung volume minus the residual volume, representing the patient's maximum breathing ability.

The relationships between these volumes and capcities are shown in Fig. 2-2.

These volumes and capacities can be measured through the use of pulmonary function tests, studies which are quite useful in the management of patients with acute and chronic pulmonary problems. A full discussion of pulmonary function testing is beyond the scope of this book. We'll concentrate on those volumes which will give you greater understanding of how to ventilate a patient.

Functional Residual Capacity

Functional Residual Capacity, or FRC, is an important concept, since this

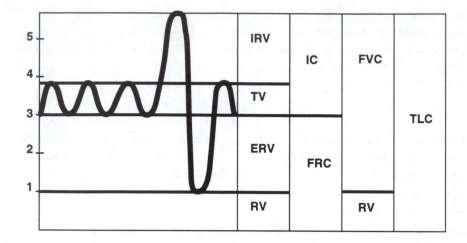

Fig. 2-2. Lung volumes and capacities in a 20-year-old male.

represents the combined gas volumes which provide most of the normal functional oxygen exchange in the lungs. The larger the FRC, the bigger the patient's "oxygen tank." A small child, who has a smaller FRC than an adult, can't hold his breathe as long without getting hypoxic.

Position also changes the FRC. An awake adult who lies supine loses about a liter of FRC as the diaphragms are pushed upward about 4 cm by the abdominal contents. The diaphragms become more concave. This diaphragmatic shape allows them to contract more with inhalation. The increased contraction produces a larger tidal volume and the patient naturally takes a deeper breath as the result. The patient with marginal respiratory reserve or morbid obesity may feel short of breath in the supine position because he can't compensate for the decreased FRC.

Induction of anesthesia, and presumably unconsciousness, further decrease FRC by approximately 0.4 liters as the diaphragm moves still higher. Hypoventilation can occur with spontanous ventilation if respiratory rate or tidal volume don't increase to compensate.

Manual ventilation changes the efficiency of this system. Now, when you squeeze the bag, the fact that the diaphragms are higher acts as a disadvantage. You must now use enough pressure to force them and the abdominal contents underneath them down and out of the way. You also have to lift the chest wall. If ventilation is difficult and vital signs allow, placing the patient 45 degrees head up will drop the abdominal contents away from the diaphragm and make lung inflation easier.

Assisting a patient who is breathing spontaneously is easier because the diaphragm continues to contract, pushing the abdominal contents down and starting the inhalation. The intercostals contract, expanding the chest wall. It's important when you assist the ventilation of a spontaneously breathing patient that you time your manual breath with his own inhalation to take advantage of this situation. What you're trying to do is augment the spontaneous breath. Ventilating while the patient is exhaling means that your inflation pressure must not only overcome the diaphragm, but reverse the passive outflow of air, the elastic recoil of the lungs, and the rebound of the chest wall combined. It usually makes the patient cough.

Tidal Volume

Tidal volume is another important concept. The average tidal volume is 7 – 8 cc/kg, for both children and adults. A normal deep breath usually equals 10 – 15 cc/kg. It's important to know the appropriate size of a patient's tidal volume. In a child, for example, giving a much larger tidal volume than normal can over pressurize the lungs and cause pneumothorax.

The tidal volume numbers noted above are for ideal body weight. A 152 cm (5'0") obese patient who weighs 120 kg (260 lb) probably won't tolerate a tidal volume of 1 liter without the risk of pneumothorax. This patient's expected maximum tidal volume, for an ideal body weight of 45 kg (99 lb), would normally be 400 – 500 cc. On the other hand, due to her obesity or clinical status, she may require more ventilation than an average adult. The way to compensate for this patient is to increase the ventilatory rate, not to increase the tidal volume.

Too small a tidal volume places the patient at risk for hypoventilation, especially if the tidal volume is smaller than or close to the volume for the patient's dead space.

Dead Space

Dead space is the portion of the tidal volume which never reaches the alveoli and is essentially wasted. It's a combination of anatomic and physiologic dead space. Anatomic dead space consists of the conducting airways such as the trachea, bronchi, and bronchioles. It's called anatomic because it's fixed by the anatomy and doesn't change. It's roughly equal in milliliters to the patient's ideal body weight in pounds or a little more than twice the body weight in kg. Thus a patient weighing 81 kg (180 lb) will have a dead space of about 180 ml. Give this 81 kg patient a tidal volume of 150 ml and you won't ventilate his alveoli very well at all. The patient will become hypercarbic and possibly hypoxic.

Physiologic dead space consists of alveoli which are ventilated but which have no capillary blood flow to pick up the oxygen and drop off carbon dioxide. In other words they are not perfused. Physiologic dead space can change depending upon the status and existing pathology of the patient. For example, pulmonary emboli obstruct the blood flow to certain sections of the lung, increasing dead space. Dead space is also increased in patients with emphysema, where the number of capillary containing alveolar septi is decreased due to enlargement of the alveoli themselves. Hypovolemia and shock can also increase physiologic dead space through the re-distribution of blood flow throughout the lungs caused by low blood pressure.

A patient with significantly increased dead space will either need a higher FiO_2, a larger tidal volume, or a faster respiratory rate to compensate.

Shunt

Unventilated alveoli which continue to be perfused by capillaries contribute to a phenomenon called shunt. This unoxygenated blood returns to the heart from the lungs and mixes with oxygenated blood. The mixture lowers the total oxygen content of the arterial blood. The presence of shunt produces hypoxemia. Give a patient with an intrapulmonary shunt 100% oxygen to breathe and the P_aO_2 won't tend to rise very much at all. The extra oxygen can't compensate for the unoxygenated blood mixing with it.

Less common anatomic causes of shunt include pulmonary arterio-venous fistulas in the lung and defects in the heart which allow mixing of oxygenated and unoxygenated blood through the septa. More common causes of shunt, however, are atelectasis, infection, pulmonary edema, and tissue trauma.

Atelectasis is the presence of collapsed alveoli. This can occur either because the alveoli failed to expand to begin with or due to the fact that the air was absorbed out of the alveoli without replacing it. To prevent atelectasis, the average person takes a very deep breath, called a sigh, several times an hour — often without even being aware of it. Patient's who take very shallow breaths without sighing often develop atelectasis.

Important risk factors for atelectasis are painful breathing, from surgery or trauma; from depressed level of consciousness from drugs; or from the disease process itself. Another less common risk factor is to allow the patient to breathe 100% oxygen. The presence of nitrogen in the alveoli helps to "splint" them open in the event that the alveolus is only intermittantly ventilated. With 100% oxygen, all of the oxygen may be easily absorbed leaving an empty alveolus. A partially inflated alveolus is easier to inflate further than a deflated alveolus. Think again of blowing up a flat balloon versus a balloon with air already in it.

When manually ventilating a patient, either with a ventilation bag or a ventilator, its important to give appropriate tidal volumes and to give the patient several "sighs" an hour to periodically maximally expand all alveoli.

Pneumonia and pulmonary edema cause shunting because some alveoli are at least partially filled with fluid. Lung tissue trauma also allows fluid into the alveoli and promotes swelling of the alveolar septi. The fluid and swelling interfere with gas diffusion.

Ventilation versus Blood Flow: V/Q Mismatch

Efficient oxygenation and elimination of carbon dioxide depends on adequate blood flow past ventilated alveoli. When the proper balance is lost, ventilation/perfusion mismatch is said to exist. The ventilation/perfusion ratio is often abbreviated **V/Q**.

Alveoli which are ventilated, but not perfused, contribute to dead space. Alveoli which are perfused, but not ventilated, contribute to shunt. Both can lead to hypoxemia and hypercarbia.

Ventilation

In the upright lung, gravity produces a pressure gradient, which causes some alveoli to be more compliant and therefore more easily inflated, than others. Because gravity causes the lung to sag toward the bottom of the chest cavity, the more dependent part of the lung is denser than the upper. The alveoli there are smaller. The alveoli at the upper parts of the lung are about four times more inflated. Picture each alveolus as a balloon. During inspiration, the smaller, dependent alveoli will be able to accept more air than the already nearly full upper alveoli. The dependent alveoli will have more air exchange and will therefore be better ventilated.

Perfusion

Distribution of the blood in the lungs is controlled by 2 factors: pulmonary artery pressure compared to intra-pulmonary air pressure; and gravity. In the upright lung, as the right ventricle beats, it sends blood into the pulmonary arteries where it then flows into the pulmonary vascular bed. As it rises, gravity slows its ascent and kinetic energy is lost. Pulmonary arterial pressure (Ppa) decreases about 1 cm H_2O per cm vertical lung distance it climbs. Ultimately Ppa becomes zero (atmospheric) and then negative (sub-atmospheric) the higher one goes.

On the other hand, the pressure inside the alveoli (P_A) remains constant independent of lung location and gravity. Three different lung zones exist because of these effects.

Zone 1 can be found in the uppermost regions of the lung. Here, the capillaries are poorly perfused because alveolar air pressure is often higher than pulmonary arterial pressure. The capillaries are collapsed. In normal lungs this rarely occurs. Zone 1 appears or increases in hypotension and shock, because pulmonary arterial pressure critically decreases compared to P_A. Increased alveolar pressure, such as from positive pressure ventilation, also increases Zone 1. In fact, in the patient in shock, providing high pressure ventilation can worsen hypotension because the alveolar filling pressure is now interfering with venous return from the lungs by impairing capillary outflow. If the patient is on a ventilator, switching to manual ventilation will often decrease pulmonary filling pressure and will help raise blood pressure.

Zone 2 lies in the middle lung regions. Here Ppa is above P_A only some of the time. Perfusion is driven by the difference between arterial pressure and the alveolar pressure (Ppa - P_A) instead of the usual difference between arterial and venous pressures. The lower in the lung one goes, the higher Ppa becomes and the better the perfusion until finally *Zone 3* is reached. In Zone 3, near the bottom of the lungs, perfusion is controlled by conventional arterial/venous pressure differences.

Near the top of the lung the alveoli are slightly over-ventilated and near the bottom of the lung the alveoli are slightly over-perfused. For the most part in the normal lung V/Q is fairly well matched.

For example, when an awake patient lies on her side, the abdominal contents push the lower, dependent diaphragm higher into the chest cavity than the upper diaphragm. The dependent diaphragm is more concave as the result. The upper is flatter. In addition, the alveoli in the dependent lung are smaller, and therefore have more room to expand than the more fully inflated upper alveoli. Thus, when the dependent diaphragm contracts, the dependent lung expands more than the upper lung. Because of gravity, blood flow to the dependent lung is also greater. Ventilation/perfusion remain matched.

If the patient loses consciousness, her FRC decreases further. Her dependent alveoli lose volume and are harder to inflate. This is similar to a deflated balloon that requires significant opening pressure to start the inflation process.

What happens when this patient must be manually ventilated on her side? Now, the more concave dependent diaphragm is a liability to push out of the way. In addition, the heart and mediastinum is resting on the dependent lung as a passive weight impeding inflation. Ventilation is more likely to go to the upper lung. Perfusion is still preferentially pulled by gravity to the dependent lung. V/Q mismatch appears. Depending on the patient's condition, this may or may not be clinically significant.

Avoiding the need for high pulmonary filling pressures when possible and maintaining adequate blood flow are essential to minimizing V/Q mismatch. If high filling pressures are needed, you may need to ensure higher blood pressures or cardiac outputs to compensate.

Intubation Criteria

Not every patient in respiratory distress needs to be intubated. The main reasons for intubation are:

- ventilatory support
- maintaining an unobstructed airway
- protection of the airway
- tracheal toilet
- elective intubation for surgery

Intubation has advantages. The tube helps protect the airway from aspiration. It permits positive pressure ventilation with 100% oxygen. It permits tracheal suctioning. It avoids the gastric distention of other techniques such as bag and mask. And it maintains an open airway in the face of edema or other fixed obstruction.

However intubation has disadvantages as well. It requires instrumentation of the airway, which can be a risk if there is potential cervical spine injury. Gagging, vomiting and aspiration can occur, especially in the conscious or semi-conscious patient. The stimulus of intubation can cause hypertension, tachycardia, and other arrythmias. In predisposed patients, the stimulus can precipitate increased intracranial pressure or myocardial ischemia. Inadvertent esophageal or mainstem intubation can occur. Finally, it's easy to forget to ventilate and oxygenate during a prolonged and difficult intubation attempt.

Ventilatory Support

The health care provider must assess the patient's clinical status and determine the most likely cause of the patient's distress. Hypoventilation and hypoxemia can occur for many reasons including:

- depression of the respiratory center by drugs;
- abnormalities of the midbrain including hemorrhage, infection, damage, or tumor;
- abnormalities of the peripheral nervous system including spinal cord injury, polio;
- diseases of the respiratory muscles including Guillain-Barre Syndrome;
- diseases of the myoneural junction such as myasthenia gravis or poisoning by certain anticholinesterase insecticides;
- trauma to the chest wall;
- damage, inflammation, infection, or collapse of a lung
- upper airway obstruction.

Ask yourself the following questions.

Is this distress caused by a condition which can be quickly reversed or improved with short term management? Is there any treatment which will rapidly improve the patient's ability to ventilate and oxygenate? Agents often used to improve a patient's respiratory status include bronchodilators for bronchospasm, diuretics for pulmonary edema, antibiotics for infection, and, of course, oxygen for support. Naloxone can reverse narcotic induced respiratory depression. A chest tube can be curative in the presence of pneumothorax. Start therapy to treat the problem.

What are the rate, depth, and pattern of respirations? Is the breathing labored?

Is there cyanosis? Cyanosis — when present — means hypoxia, and it must be treated aggressively. On the other hand, the patient can be hypoxic but not cyanotic. To be able to see the skin color change of cyanosis there has to be at least 5 gm% of desaturated Hgb in the tissues. If the patient is very anemic, cyanosis may be absent. It may also be difficult to assess a patient for cyanosis when he has darker skin tones or is in a dim environment.

Can the patient maintain an O_2 sat of at least 90% or a PaO_2 of at least 60 mmHg on less than 50% FiO_2? These values will provide the minimum oxygen content in a patient with a normal Hgb to deliver enough oxygen to the tissues. You may need to maintain a higher O_2 sat and PaO_2 if the patient is anemic.

Do you expect the disease process causing the hypoxia or hypoventilation to persist or progress?

Does the patient show signs of exhaustion? An exhausted patient is frequently losing the battle to compensate for his illness.

If you have access to blood gas results, what do they show? How abnormal are they? Patients in respiratory distress often hyperventilate to compensate. The $PaCO_2$ is low and the pH higher than normal. If a patient in severe respiratory distress has a normal pH and $PaCO_2$ this is a dangerous sign. It means that the patient is exhausted and will soon begin to hypoventilate. If the patient in distress has an acidic pH and a high $PaCO_2$, then the patient has decompensated and needs some form of respiratory support.

Is there serious cardiovascular instability? Shock from any cause can precipitate hypoventilation and hypoxia and in turn can be made worse by hypoventilation and hypoxia. If the situation is deteriorating, intubating the airway for more secure airway control may help to stabilize the situation.

Will you be able to monitor the patient at high risk for serious respiratory failure closely for further decompensation? If the answer to this question is no, then you should consider intubation.

Maintaining an Unobstructed Airway

Airway obstruction can occur due to the presence of a foreign body, loss of muscle tone, bleeding, and edema. It can be mild or life-threatening. Patients at risk for developing airway obstruction include those with trauma, infection, burns, allergic reactions, or altered consciousness. Any patient may be at potential risk of airway obstruction.

Evaluating the degree of airway obstruction is a judgement call.

Mild or potential obstruction may have no signs or symptoms at all. The patient may have a slight cough or mild hoarseness.

With moderate obstruction, the patient will have stridor on slight exertion. **Stridor** is noisy breathing caused by the increased turbulence of air moving past an obstruction. Rib retraction on inspiration and dilation of the nostrils appears. The patient uses his accessory muscles of respiration. You will see indrawing of the cervical soft tissue and a tracheal "tug." The patient will often complain of dyspnea.

In severe obstruction the patient will often have stridor at rest. Be careful, however. If air exchange is minimal there may be no stridor at all. The patient will begin to show signs of hypoxia: apprehension, restlessness, sweating, pallor, tachycardia, hypertension. You will see exaggerated neck vein filling with respirations.

When obstruction becomes severe enough, you'll see slowed respirations, hypotension, cyanosis, and impaired consciousness. Once the patient reaches this stage, cardiac arrest is imminent. You must act immediately.

In certain patients such as facial burn victims, mild airway obstruction can convert to total obstruction quickly as edema forms. It's often better to secure the airway early in these patients rather than wait.

Techniques for managing airway obstruction are covered in Chapter 3.

Protection of the Airway

A patient with altered levels of consiousness may have a depressed gag reflex and be unable to protect his airway from aspiration. Trauma victims and patients in shock are at high risk of vomiting due to gastro-intestinal tract dysfunction. Securing the airway for protection in these patients can be life-saving.

Tracheal Toilet

Occasionally a patient won't be able to clear secretions from the tracheobronchial tree by coughing. For example, a patient with end-stage chronic obstructive pulmonary disease with pneumonia may need intubation to allow suctioning of the secretions to allow the patient to recover.

The criteria for intubation in trauma victims will be futher discussed in Chapter 12.

Managing the airway requires ongoing assessment of both the airway and the total patient status. Some knowledge of physiology gives you better understanding of the reasons behind your actions. Such knowledge makes you better able to adapt your treatment plans in quickly changing clinical situations.

3 ESTABLISHING AN AIRWAY

Opening an obstructed airway is a different skill from intubation, but the two are inseparable. The ability to ventilate a patient is often more important than the ability to intubate a patient and should be learned first. Intubation is merely one means of ventilating and protecting the airway. Rarely will intubation — by itself — save a life. Ventilation, on the other hand, frequently saves lives.

Recognizing Airway Obstruction

Examine the patient for signs of airway obstruction (Table 3–1).

Is there air exchange? Is the chest moving and how much? Are both sides of the chest expanding equally? Place your hand over the nose or mouth and feel if

---

Table 3-1. Evidence of Airway Obstruction

- poor movement of air
- faint or absent breath sounds
- stridor
- use of accessory muscles of respiration
- tracheal tug
- space between ribs sucked inward
- rocking chest motion: chest falls and the abdomen rises on inspiration
- cyanosis

---

there is air movement. When wearing gloves you can use the back of your hand or wrist. If there is a clear oxygen mask over the face look for condensation with exhalation. Does the tidal volume seem adequate?

Listen to the chest bilaterally for the presence of breath sounds. At the same time listen to their quality. Do you hear upper airway noises compatible with obstruction? Are breath sounds equal? Are there rales or wheezes?

Is there stridor? Stridor is the harsh, creaking, noisy respiration produced by air turbulence when the airway is partially obstructed. Snoring is also a sign of obstruction.

When the patient is working hard to breathe, the accessory muscles of respiration — the sternocleidomastoid and scalene neck muscles — tense as though the patient is straining. These muscles lift the clavicles and allow fuller expansion of the chest.

When the patient works harder to take a breath, a greater vacuum is generated inside the chest cavity. This effort is seen on the outside as a tracheal tug, where the soft tissue at the top of the sternum is sucked inward. The space between the ribs is also sucked inward.

A rocking chest motion is usually apparent, with the abdomen rising and the chest falling as the patient inhales. This occurs as the diaphragm descends maximally, pushing out the abdominal contents and generating increased vacuum. With airway obstruction, no air can enter the chest, so the chest wall falls in response.

If inadequate ventilation persists long enough, cyanosis develops. Cyanosis is a late sign which is often hard to see depending on ambient lighting, patient skin tone, and the presence of severe anemia.

Opening the Airway

If the patient is apneic proceed immediately to ventilate him or her with a bag and a mask. On the other hand, if the patient is breathing spontaneously, but is obstructed, there are several ways to open the airway.

The easiest is to grab the mandible behind each jaw angle and lift. Also, extend the head if there is no risk of cervical spine injury. Both maneuvers pull the tongue and associated structures upward and usually relieve the obstruction (Fig. 3-1a-d, 3-2a, b). Because pressing on the angle of the jaw is painful, this maneuver often has the benefit of waking a stuporous patient — another means of improving the airway.

If you still have a marginal airway insert a nasal or an oral airway. See Table 3-1 for the signs of airway obstruction.

Terminology can be confusing. Not only do we call the patient's passageway from mouth to trachea an airway, we also call the tools to establish an open breathing passage airways. Context usually makes the meaning clear.

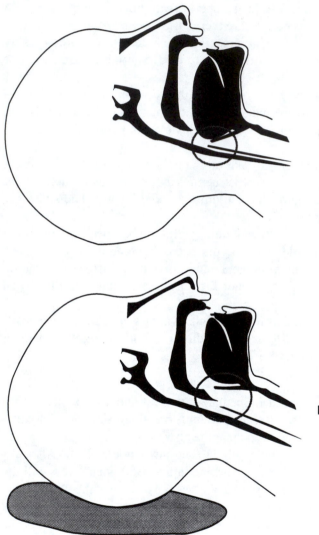

a. OBSTRUCTED AIRWAY

b. SNIFFING POSITION

Fig. 3-1a,b. Opening an obstructed airway.

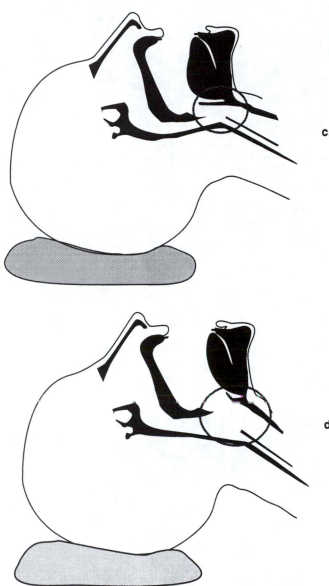

c. TILT HEAD BACK

d. PULL THE ANGLES
OF THE JAW UPWARD

Fig. 3-1c,d. Opening an obstructed airway.

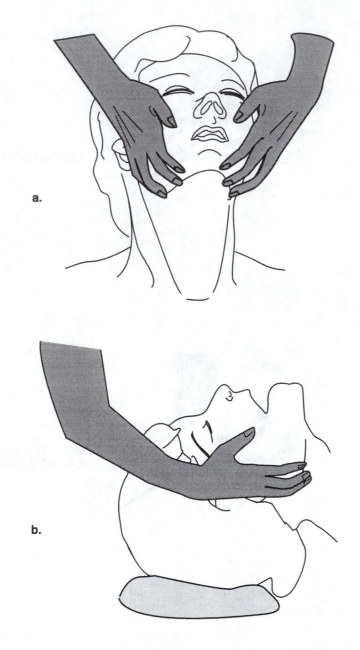

a.

b.

Fig. 3-2a,b. To open the airway, extend the head and thrust the jaw forward.

Use of the Nasal Airway

Nasal airways, also called nasal cannulas, are soft, flexible tubes which slide through one side of the nose. This positions the opening of the tube in the posterior pharynx, behind the tongue. The opening is often, though not always, in line with the trachea.

Awake patients often tolerate a nasal airway better than an oral airway because it stimulates the gag reflex less. Liberally coat your nasal airway with some lubricating ointment if available. Local anesthetic ointment has the advantage of numbing the nose and making the tube more easily tolerated. However, water or non-anesthetic jelly works as well. Slide the nasal airway into the nares and gently advance it along the floor of the nose (Fig. 3-3a, b). The beginner will frequently try to thread the nasal airway up the nose toward the frontal

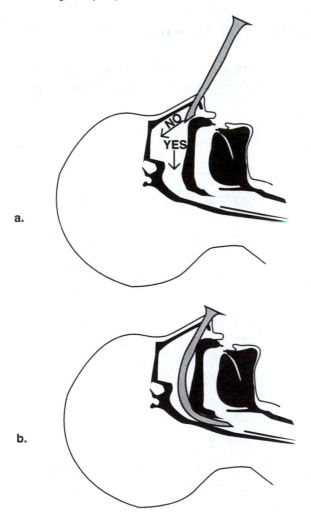

a.

b.

Fig. 3-3a,b. Direct the nasal airway along the floor of the nose. Slide it forward to position it in the posterior pharynx.

sinus. Not only will the tube not pass in this direction, you risk a nose bleed. If you meet an obstruction then carefully twist the tube while slowly pushing it forward. Don't force it. The turbinates can be fragile and easily fractured and the mucosa is easily torn. Check your angle of insertion and try again. If the nasal airway will not pass, try the other nares or switch to a smaller tube.

The nasal passage sometimes pinches the tube as it turns the corner. This may make suctioning down the nasal airway difficult because the narrowing may prevent passage of a suction catheter.

You can use a nasal airway to ventilate any patient when ventilation with a bag and a mask is difficult. Simply insert an endotracheal tube connector into the nasal end of a nasal airway. Choose one that fits snugly. The nasal airway will now connect to your ventilation circuit. Hold the mouth and opposite nostril firmly closed. Squeezing the bag will now ventilate the patient (Fig. 3-4).

Use of the Oral Airway

An oral airway is a fairly firm, curved piece of plastic. It sits on top of the tongue and pulls the tongue and associated structures forward. Oral airways have several disadvantages.

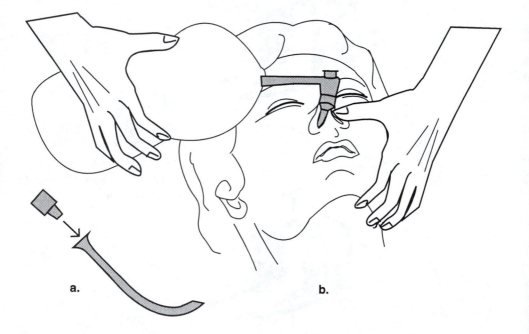

a.   b.

Fig. 3-4a, b. An alternate means of ventilation — insert an endotracheal tube connector into a nasal airway as in **a.** Place the nasal airway, close the opposite nostril and mouth. Ventilate as in **b.**

First, the oral airway must be placed inside the mouth between the patient's teeth, sometimes a difficult and personally risky task in awake patients who are protecting their airway. Never place your unprotected fingers inside a patient's mouth unless you're fairly certain that he or she can't bite you. Fortunately, there are several ways of inserting oral airways without having to so this.

Second, firm, plastic oral airways can damage teeth — especially if the teeth are already loose or decayed.

Third, the tip of the oral airway sits on the back of the tongue. An awake patient will sometimes gag, vomit and possibly aspirate. This is especially true if the patient's mental status is compromised.

Having stated the disadvantages, let me also state that oral airways relieve most types of obstruction very effectively. They are one of our most important tools. The correct size oral airway places the flange immediately outside the teeth or gums and positions the tip near the vallecula. To estimate the correct size, place the airway next to the patient's jaw parallel to the mouth and judge where it will lie. Too small an airway places the tip in the middle of the tongue. This bunches the tissue and worsens obstruction. Too large an airway will extend from the mouth and prevent sealing the mask over the face.

There are several ways to insert an oral airway. Open the mouth widely, as you would to intubate the patient. Insert the oral airway with the curve either down toward the tongue, or up toward the roof of the mouth. With the curve down, advance the airway until the tip is behind the back of the tongue. Properly placed the airway pulls the tongue forward. Improperly placed it pushes the tongue into the back of the pharynx and further obstructs the airway. Wetting the airway with water will allow it to slide more easily.

You can use a tongue blade in the left hand to help open the mouth and push the tongue down. Place the tongue blade to the rear of the tongue and pull it forward. Often this allows you to slide the oral airway in without any further problem (3-5a, b). At this point, if I still can't insert the airway, I grasp it firmly in my right hand and force it to straighten as much as possible (Fig. 3-6a, b). I then place the straightened airway on the tongue blade and slide it down the blade to the back of the mouth. Once in position I relax my grip. The oral airway springs back into its curve and pulls the tongue forward.

Many people insert an oral airway by turning its curve toward the roof of the mouth. They advance it until its tip lies behind the tongue and then flip the airway into position (Fig. 3-7a, b). While very effective, you must use caution. You can easily damage teeth and the roof of the mouth, especially if the mouth is not wide open.

Ventilating with a Bag and a Mask

Having established the airway you should next check ventilation. If the patient is breathing adequately, you can decide the need for intubation and for such treatments as narcotic reversal with less haste. Apply oxygen by mask while you do this. If the patient is not breathing well you must immediately assist or control his respiration. Both require the use of some form of bag and mask apparatus.

For the bag and mask to work you must have a good seal on the mask. This means pressing the mask against the patient's face to effectively prevent the escape of the pressurized breaths you deliver.

First, choose the correct size mask for the patient. Most women take a small mask. Most men will use a medium. Tall men may need a large. Large children

TONGUE BLADE   **ORAL AIRWAY**

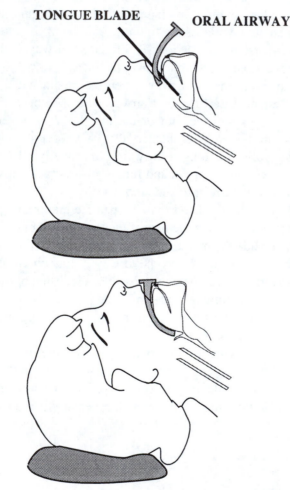

a.

b.

Fig. 3-5a,b. Push tongue down with tongue blade, then slide the oral airway into position.

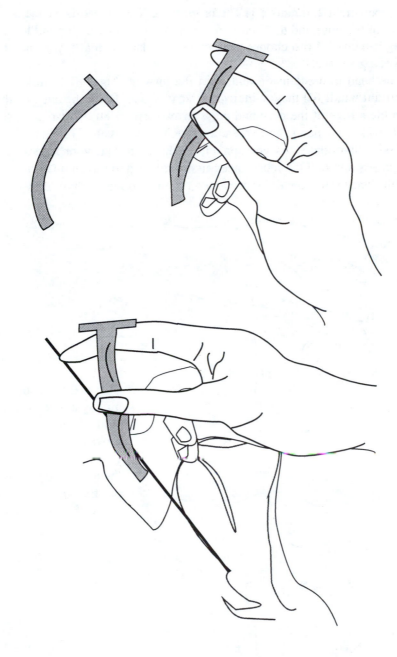

Fig. 3-6. Straighten the oral airway with your fingers, then slide it down the tongue blade until the tip is behind the tongue.

need a 3, toddlers a 2, infants a 1. The proper size just covers the space between the bridge of the nose and the crease in the chin. The entire upper and lower lips fit inside the mask. If you choose too small or too large a mask, you may find it hard to get a good seal.

Pull the head into extension and open the airway (Fig. 3-8a). Hold it there with your left hand. All masks are triangular in shape. Place the apex of the triangle on the bridge of the nose and press firmly (Fig. 3-8b). Grasp each side of the mask with your hands and spread as much as you can. This is easier with some masks than others. As you spread, reach down with your free index and middle fingers and pull the loose cheek tissue forward to bunch on either side of the mouth. Place your remaining fingers on the jaw bone and pull upward. This

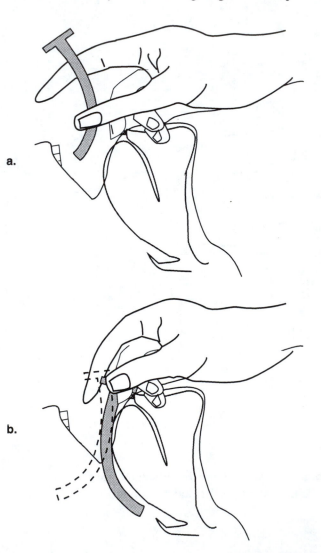

a.

b.

Fig. 3-7. Insert the airway upside down. When flipping the airway, make sure that you avoid pressure on the upper teeth. The hard plastic can also scrape the roof of the mouth.

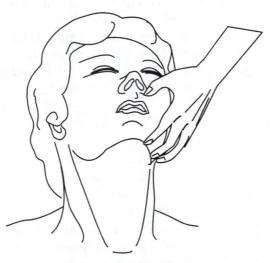

a.   **Extend the head to open the airway.**

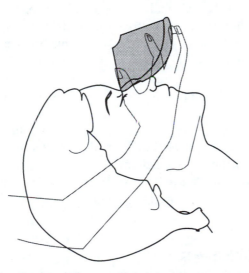

b.   **Masks have a triangular shape. Place the apex of the triangle
over the bridge of the nose.**

Fig. 3-8a, b. Getting a good mask seal. (See following page for
more.)

action also holds the head in extension and holds the airway open while you position the mask. Now, lower the mask over the cheeks and allow the edges to grab the bunched cheek tissue (Fig. 3-8c, d). Make sure the lower lip is inside the mask. Take your right hand off the mask and maintain your seal and jaw lift with the left (Fig. 3-9). Squeeze the bag with your right hand. If you have a good seal no air will escape around the mask. You can tolerate some leak as long as you can ventilate the patient. If not, you must get a better fit.

The extra bulk of the bunched cheek tissue fills in the gaps between the mask and the patient and helps seal it. In certain patients, especially edentulous ones, this may not work. Typically the mask leaks on the side opposite the hand holding the mask. First, use the weight of the bag on the leaky side to force the mask against the patient's face. If this doesn't work, then place gauze in the gap to seal the hole. Alternatively, you can ask a helper to push the cheek up against the outside of the mask at the leak sites. This seals the hole very effectively. Once again use your helpers if you have problems.

The ability to ventilate is the ultimate test of success in positioning both patient and equipment. Squeeze the bag. The chest should rise with each breath. Have a helper listen to the chest to verify breath sounds as you ventilate. As you squeeze the bag pay attention to the resistance you feel as the lungs inflate. Obstruction makes squeezing the bag difficult or impossible. A leak in the ventilation system makes squeezing the bag extremely easy. In both these cases, however, the chest won't rise. Educating your hand is valuable because it allows you to monitor your patient without staring at the chest. If you can tell how well you ventilate the patient without looking you free your attention for other matters. Don't forget that difficulty in ventilation may be due to your patient's illness and not to your technique. Congestive heart failure, bronchospasm, and pneumothorax can also make airway resistance worse, breath sounds fainter, and ventilation difficult. You must prove, however, that the fault is not your own before blaming poor ventilation on the patient.

Placing oral or nasal airways at this point may improve your ventilation if you have not already done so. Suction the secretions, if any, to prevent aspiration.

Optimal Use of the Self-Inflating Bag

The use of a self-inflating bag without supplemental oxygen will deliver an oxygen concentration of 21%. Most sick or injured patients need more than this. When the bag is attached to oxygen at a rate of 10–12 liters per minute you will deliver oxygen levels of 40–60%. Adding a reservoir bag and running the oxygen at 12–15 liters per minute raises the concentration to 100%, but only if the reservoir is allowed to fill.

When using a self-inflating bag it's important to squeeze the bag in a manner designed to maximize oxygen concentration. When you abruptly allow the bag

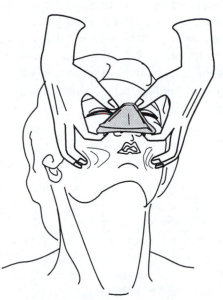

c.   Hold mask top against bridge of nose. Spread sides with hands. Push cheek tissue under mask edges.

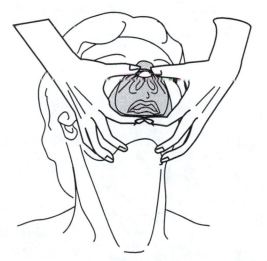

d.   Lower mask over cheeks. Let edges grab bunched tissue. Seat over chin. Make sure lower lip is inside mask.

Fig. 3-8c, d. Getting a good mask seal.

to refill after squeezing it, it will tend to refill with room air rather than with oxygen, whose inflow is time limited. It is better to allow the bag to refill over 3–4 seconds by releasing the pressure of your hand gradually over that time period.

Your left hand holding the mask will tend to tire quickly if you keep it constantly tensed. Fatigue then interferes with your ability to ventilate. Learn to maintain the mask seal using the least amount of tension in your hands as possible. Relax the left hand slightly as the bag refills. This technique will allow you to ventilate for prolonged periods of time.

Difficult Ventilation

Obese Patients

Large or fat patients occasionally force you to use both hands to seal the mask. Excess soft tissue collapsing over the laryngeal structures may make manual ventilation difficult. Try placing an oral or nasal airway if you have trouble ventilating this type of patient. Frequently this is all you need to do. Ask for an assistant if obstruction persists. Use both of your hands to obtain a good seal on the mask (Fig. 3-10). Place one hand on either side of the head. Place your thumbs at the top of the mask and hold the bottom of the mask down forcefully with your index fingers. Pull the jaw upward with your remaining fingers by spreading them along the jaw line, underneath the angle of the mandible. The basic hand position is the same as that just described. Pull up forcefully. Hold just the bone. Pushing on the soft tissue under the jaw can force it into the airway and worsen obstruction.

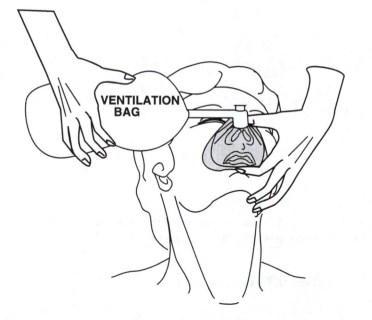

Fig. 3-9. Holding the mask while squeezing the bag.

With this movement you shift the mandible forward and pull the obstructing tissue up and off the larynx. Your assistant can now squeeze the ventilation bag. Move your fingers as needed to perfect your seal. Even when using both hands on the mask, you may need a helper to stop the leaks. When using this technique, be sure that your assistant is adequately ventilating the patient. Watch the chest rise, see the air condense on the mask if it is clear, and have someone listen for breath sounds.

Manual ventilation can be very difficult in the obese patient or the patient with increased intra-abdominal pressure. It can limit the ability to deliver an adequate tidal volume. Placing this type of patient in reverse trendelenburg allows the abdominal contents to drop away from the diaphragm and lowers the amount of pressure needed to deliver the breath.

Edentulous Patients

Ventilation of the edentulous patient can cause problems. Sealing the mask without the teeth to give support to the cheeks and form to the mouth is challenging. I find the newer, low dead space masks with an inflated cuff around the edge easiest to use. They conform to the loose contour of the face with less tendency to allow gaps and air leaks. However, even these masks occasionally fail.

When gaps occur they are usually over the bridge of the nose or on the side opposite the hand holding the mask. With the left hand holding the mask, the leak usually appears on the right side. First, simply allow the weight of your

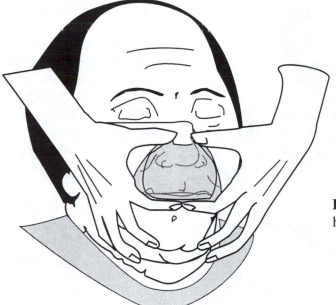

Fig. 3-10. Using both hands to seal the mask.

ventilation bag and attachments to push down the mask help obtain a seal. Turn the apparatus on the connector until its weight is centered over the leak. If this doesn't work, try plugging the leak with a piece of gauze under the mask. An assistant can help push cheek tissue up over the mask edge at the site of the leak or leaks.

If the above fails, try a variation on the two handed technique I described for the obese patient (Fig.3-10). Place your thumbs on the top of the mask, your index fingers on the bottom. Use your middle and ring fingers to bunch the cheek tissue up to seal the mask on either side. This leaves your fifth fingers free to hook under the mandible and lift. Your assistant ventilates.

You can use the weight of your own chin over the bridge of the mask to stop leaks here (Fig. 3-11). While the position sounds awkward, it does allow you to ventilate the patient fairly well. I often use it in the absence of assistants to help me.

Another trick consists of placing an infant-sized Rendall-Baker mask in the patient's mouth — under the cheeks but outside the gums. This recreates the form and support of the missing teeth. The mask fits over the mouth and cheeks without leaks. The hole in the pediatric mask lets you ventilate (Fig. 3-12).

Poor Compliance

Compliance is a term used to describe how easy it is to inflate the patient's lungs. Poor compliance can be caused by many conditions including:

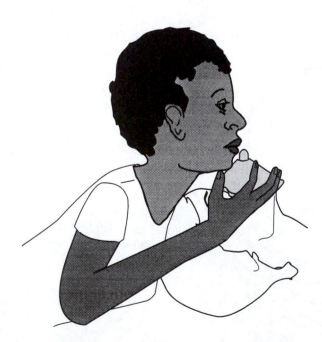

Fig. 3-11. One technique to maintain a good seal with a leak over the nose. In the absence of helpers pressure from your own chin can press the mask down over the nose. One hand helps seal. The other one ventilates the patient as needed.

- compression of the lungs, such as pneumothorax or hemothorax;
- change in lung tissue consistency, such as pulmonary edema;
- change in airway resistance, such as bronchospasm;
- increased intra-abdominal pressure, such as pregnancy, obesity, distended stomach;
- chest wall rigidity, from certain drugs or from muscle spasm.

Regardless of the cause, manual ventilation may be difficult. Make sure that you have a good mask seal and an open airway. You will be needing to use higher inflation pressures. If the airway is not open the air will tend to take the path of least resistance and enter the stomach, predisposing to vomiting and perhaps worsening compliance. You may need to decompress the stomach with a nasogastric tube when the situation permits.

If the inflation pressures are very high you may need both of your hands on the mask to effectively seal it. Your assistant will probably need both hands on the bag to deliver an adequate tidal volume. Squeeze the bag more slowly, allowing the gas time to enter. This type of patient frequently needs to be intubated at the earliest opportunity.

The ability to handle airway obstruction and to ventilate with a bag and a mask are equally as important, if not more important, than the ability to intubate. Practice at every available opportunity.

Further Reading

Lopez NR: Mechanical problems of the airway. *Clin. Anes.* 1968; 3: 8

Linscott MS, Horton WC: Management of upper airway obstruction. *Otolaryngol. Clin. North Am.* 1979; 12:351-373

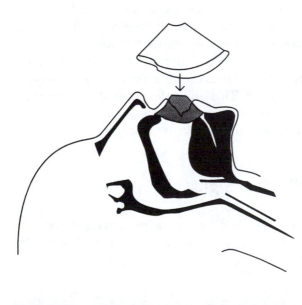

Fig. 3-12. In edentulous patients you can place an infant mask inside the cheeks on top of the gums. An adult mask fits over the cheeks and usually seals well.

4 PREINTUBATION EVALUATION: PREDICTING THE DIFFICULT AIRWAY

A simple medical history and physical exam will often alert you to potential problems with intubation and airway management. Such forwarning allows you to alter your technique and your equipment from the start. In the elective situation this is no problem.

The emergency situation is more difficult because you won't have the luxury of a prolonged evaluation and leisurely analysis. Fortunately, you can easily spot many of the warning signs of a difficult airway. Additionally, medical care providers at scenes of emergencies can tell you important information if you know what to ask. This rapid analysis lets you rationally choose endotracheal tube size, type and size of laryngoscope blade, and technique.

Medical History

Operations in and around the airway can produce distortion by either changing or removing normal anatomical landmarks. Recent surgery, trauma, tumor, and infection often produce edema or hematoma formation. These not only distort the landmarks but can cause airway obstruction. Nasal fractures often deviate the septum, causing a problem with nasal intubation. Past surgery or irradiation of the neck create scar tissue. This limits the range of motion of the larynx, fixing it in position. It can also limit the range of motion of the head and neck. Anything that alters anatomy or limits motion of the larynx or neck makes difficult intubation more likely.

Physical Signs

Short muscular or obese neck — The larynx on these patients is often higher in the neck, opposite the fourth cervical vertebrae and higher. This

60

makes it harder for the laryngoscope to push the tongue and epiglottis forward. Downward pressure on the vallecula often folds the epiglottis down, hiding the cords. This makes curved blades more difficult to use in these patients. The patient's teeth can be an added disadvantage because teeth limit your ability to maneuver the blade. These patients often require a straight blade and cricoid pressure for intubation.

Receding Chin — Patients with receding chins have hypoplastic or poorly developed mandibles. Again, there is less room to displace the tongue and epiglottis forward. Identify these patients by looking at their profile and noting the chin line. Spot them also by measuring the distance from the inside of the mandible to the hyoid bone with your fingertips. This distance is normally at least three fingers breadths in the adult (Fig. 4-1). Less than three is an indication that you may have difficulty. Two or less almost assures it. Have these patients extend their necks. A distance from the lower border of the mandible to the thyroid notch of less than 6 cm alerts you to potential problems.

Patients with receding chins and those with short necks have a so-called "anterior larynx." Their larynx isn't more anterior in their neck when seen in profile. But when you try to view their larynx with the laryngoscope, the entire structure lies anterior to your field of view (Fig. 4-2). Since the larynx is higher in the neck, there is less room to displace the other structures forward to clear

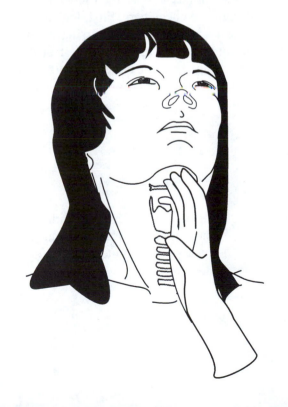

Fig. 4-1. Measuring the distance from the mentum of the chin to the hyoid bone — 3 fingers breadth in the adult.

the path to the larynx. The larynx can be very hard to see. Sometimes you only see the arytenoids. At other times you can see no landmarks at all. Straight blades and cricoid pressure should come to mind when you spot the signs.

Overbite — The presence of an overbite (the protrusion of the incisor teeth due to relative overgrowth of the premaxilla) hampers intubation. There is less room to maneuver your blade. The upper teeth simply get in the way. In these patients it is especially important to lift the mandible and extend the head as much as possible. This prevents using the teeth as a fulcrum.

Limited Mobility of the Mandible — Opening the mouth requires two movements: opening the hinge joint on a vertical axis and then sliding the angle of the jaw forward. Check both since arthritis, scar tissue, and spasm of the masseter muscle can impair either movement. First check the patient's ability to open the mouth widely (Fig. 4-3). Normally, adults can open the mouth at least three cm or about three finger breadths. When a patient can't open that broadly, it impairs your ability to maneuver and to see. You may not be able to insert your blade at all.

Second, check the ability to displace the mandible. Have the patient push his lower jaw forward to place his lower teeth in front of his upper teeth (Fig. 4-4). If he can't, you might not be able to pull the mandible forward far enough to see the larynx. Patients with temporomandibular joint arthritis frequently lose the forward glide of their jaw before they lose their ability to open their mouths.

Oral Cavity — There are a number of things to check here. First, look at the condition of the teeth. Notice teeth that are loose, chipped, or missing before you start. Look at the relative size of the tongue in relation to the rest of the mouth. Young children have relatively large tongues. Sometimes, patients with oral tumors or trauma have a swollen or enlarged tongue. High arched palates

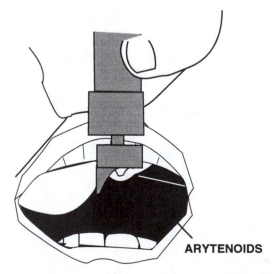

Fig. 4-2. The view seen with an anterior larynx. Here you can see the arytenoids. Often you see no landmarks.

ARYTENOIDS

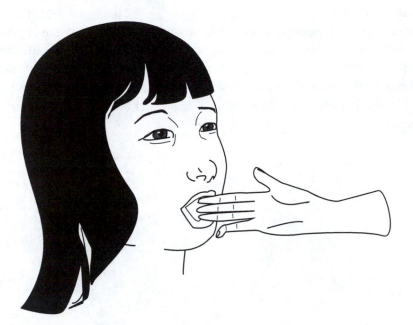

Fig. 4-3. Can the patient open his or her mouth wide enough for 3 fingers?

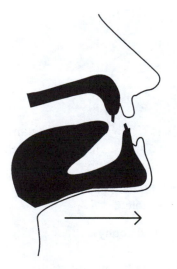

Fig. 4-4. Have the patients place their lower teeth outside their upper teeth to check for the ability of their jaw to glide forward.

with narrow mouths make passage of the tube difficult because the blade itself takes up so much room.

Finally, have the erect patient open his mouth as widely as possible and look at the posterior pharynx. You can use Mallampati's signs and classification to identify patients at risk for difficult intubation (Fig. 4-5). Visibility of intraoral structures correlates with ease of viewing with a laryngoscope. Patients in categories I and II are low risk. Patients in category III and IV are at high risk for problems.

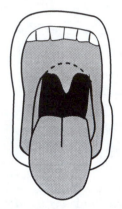

Class I: soft palate, uvula, fauces, pillars visible

No difficulty

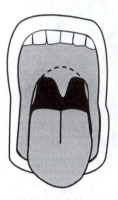

Class II: soft palate, uvula, fauces visible

No difficulty

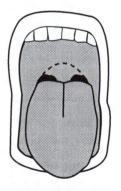

Class III: soft palate, base of uvula visible

Moderate difficulty

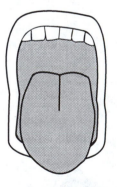

Class IV: hard palate only visible

Severe difficulty

Fig. 4-5. Mallampati Signs as indicators of difficulty of intubation. (Adapted from Mallampati and Samsoon and Young.)

Flexion and extension of the Neck — Have the patient touch his chin to his chest (normal 45°) and to both shoulders in turn (normal 40°). Then have the patient extend his head back as far as possible (normal 55°). Normal range of motion decreases about 20% by 70 years of age.

Limited range of motion impairs your ability to bring the axes into alignment. If the atlanto-occipital joint cannot fully extend, then marked extension of the head on the neck increases the anterior cervical spine convexity. This pushes the larynx further anteriorly, impairing the view.

External larynx — Look at the trachea and the external laryngeal structures. Are they midline in the neck or deviated to one side? Tumor, trauma, hematoma, and scar tissue can deviate the trachea. Movement of the larynx from the midline makes identification of landmarks and alignment of axes more difficult. Place your hand over the larynx and gently move it from side to side. A larynx fixed to the midline by tumor or scar is often hard to lift with the laryngoscope. It looks anterior and is often very hard to see (Fig. 4-6).

Vocal cords — Indirect exam of the vocal cords entails listening to the voice. The presence of hoarseness can mean edema, tumor, paralysis, or

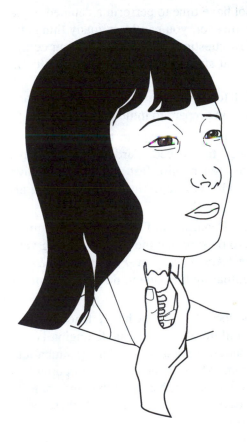

Fig. 4-6. Gently move the larynx from side to side to check for masses and immobility.

arthritis. All of the above imply the need for a smaller than average endotracheal tube. I try to place the largest tube possible for the patient — to minimize the need for excessive cuff inflation, to assist suctioning, and to minimize airway resistance. However, I will often start with a smaller tube if I expect a smaller opening. This is especially true in emergencies when I don't want to risk inability to pass the tube on the first try.

You can examine the vocal cords with an indirect laryngoscopy mirror before intubation if there is any question of possible obstruction. Special, soft tissue X-rays and other studies may also be helpful in the non-emergency situation.

Nose — Checking the nose is important if you plan a nasal intubation. Ask the patient if he has ever broken his nose. Is the septum deviated? Check to see if he can breath equally out both sides or if one side is more patent. Is there a history of nose bleeds or sinusitis, which may predispose the patient to complications from a nasal intubation?

Remember that patients who are potentially difficult to intubate may also be difficult to ventilate if given a general anesthetic. If you have any doubt about your ability to ventilate the patient, you should place the tube with the patient awake.

In the emergency situation you will not have time to perform a detailed physical exam or take an involved history. However, you can learn many things by just looking at the patient and asking a few questions as you prepare your equipment. A few well-spent minutes before you start often prevents a difficult and prolonged intubation attempt.

Let's imagine that you've been called to intubate a patient that you don't know. Ask the following questions while you prepare to intubate.

1. Why does this patient need intubation? The answer to this question will let you know how quickly you need to proceed. Cardiac arrest victims and patients dying from lack of oxygen require fast action. Progressive respiratory failure in an asthmatic who is tiring, but still ventilating, allows more time for analysis.

2. Is someone ventilating this patient? Regardless of the reason for intubation, your first duty in the room is to be sure that the patient is being ventilated and oxygenated. *Ventilation takes priority over everything else.* If you are the only one capable of ventilating the patient, do so. Have an assistant prepare your equipment.

3. What important medical problems does this patient have? Knowing that an awake patient with respiratory failure also has unstable angina is important if you are to minimize hypertension and stress during intubation. Knowing that a patient suffers from AIDS or hepatitis is important to know to protect yourself during the intubation. Nasal intubations are relatively contraindicated in immunosuppressed patients and those with diabetes because of the risk of sinusitus.

4. Is this patient anticoagulated? Intubation techniques in the anticoagulated patient must be especially gentle to prevent bleeding into the airway. Additionally, you should not perform a nasal intubation in an anticoagulated patient due to the risk of nose bleed.

5. Is there any problem with the airway? When I encounter a history of surgery, trauma, tumor, radiation or infection of the airway I reach for a straight, rather than a curved, blade and for a smaller, rather than a larger, tube.

During this exchange you are quickly choosing what you feel is the appropriate laryngoscope blade and tube. You are checking the cuff on the tube for leaks and inserting a stylet. And you are asking for suction — with a yankauer suction tip if possible. Suction is often a low priority item for the resuscitation team. It is a high priority item for you because you need to see the larynx and you need to clear the airway.

A quick look at the patient identifies such signs as a receding chin, an overbite, facial trauma, a deviated trachea, and a short, thick neck. Ventilating the patient before the intubation identifies problems with neck and jaw mobility. It took less than the 2-4 minutes you needed to prepare your equipment to do a simple evaluation of the patient's airway.

However, sometimes the tests for prediction of the difficult intubation are wrong. The likelihood of an easy intubation is high if multiple predictive tests are negative. On the other hand, you must always be prepared for the possibility that any intubation may still be difficult.

References

Benumof JL. Management of the difficult adult airway, with special emphasis on awake tracheal intubation. *Anes* 1990; 72: 1087-1110.

Cormack RS. Diffcult tracheal intubation in obstetrics. *Anaes* 1984; 39:1105-1111.

Mallampati SR, Gatt SP, Gugino LD et al..: A clinical sign to predict difficult tracheal intubation: a prospective study. Can Anaesth Soc J 1985; 32:429-434.

Samsoon GLT, Young JRB. Difficult tracheal intubation: a retrospective study: *Anes* 1987: 42:487-490.

5 Equipment

To intubate you need an endotracheal tube, and the ability to identify the larynx, suction the airway, and ventilate the patient. Most emergency settings in the United States have specialized equipment readily available. Optimally, you should have the following list of supplies.

Equipment you need for intubation includes:

- laryngoscope handle with functioning batteries
- laryngoscope blade with functioning light bulb, both straight and curved if possible
- proper sizes of endotracheal tubes
- suction apparatus, with yankauer and flexible catheters
- syringe for inflating endotracheal tube cuff
- stylet

Equipment you should have for airway management includes:

- oral airway
- nasal airway
- oxygen supply
- Magill forceps
- mask and bag ventilating apparatus
- means of securing tube, such as tape
- stethoscope for checking proper tube placement

We'll discuss the use of all the equipment later. Now let's concentrate on checking the equipment for functionality.

Checking Your Laryngoscope

First check your laryngoscope blade and handle. To attach the blade to the handle notice that the handle has a post on top — inside of a square depression. The blade has a matching hook shaped flange. Hold the handle in your left hand and the blade in your right so the flange hooks over the post and seats into the depression (Fig. 5-1a). Push the blade forward until you feel it snap into place (Fig. 5-1b). The blade will be at an angle to the handle. The fit should be snug so the blade does not fall off the handle when in the off position.

To turn the laryngoscope on, pull the blade into a right angle with the handle (Fig. 5-1c). Again you should feel a snap as it locks. The light should turn on. If it doesn't, tighten the light bulb connection. If the bulb still fails to light, change

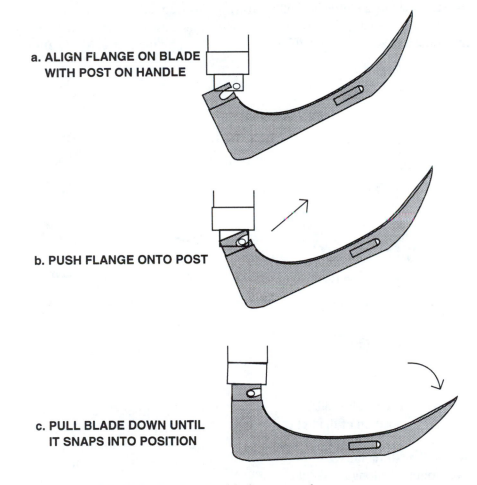

a. ALIGN FLANGE ON BLADE
WITH POST ON HANDLE

b. PUSH FLANGE ONTO POST

c. PULL BLADE DOWN UNTIL
IT SNAPS INTO POSITION

Fig. 5-1. Placing the blade on your laryngoscope.

the batteries and/or the bulb and try again. Finally, remove the blade and check the contact points between the blade and the handle. Occasionally you must clean the contacts just as you clean the contacts on a battery. Use an alcohol swab, an eraser, or an emory board. You should periodically check the intubation equipment before you need it. Trouble shooting in the middle of an emergency is inappropriate.

If you haven't done so, look at the differences between a curved and a straight blade. There are many variations of straight and curved blades. The most common ones in use are the curved MacIntosh blades and the straight Miller blades (Fig. 5-2, 5-3).

Checking Your Endotracheal Tube

Next, check the endotracheal tube cuff (Fig. 5-4). Attach your syringe, usually a ten cc syringe, to the pilot balloon and distend the cuff with air. Detach the syringe and check to see if the cuff leaks — as shown by the loss of air. Leaks can

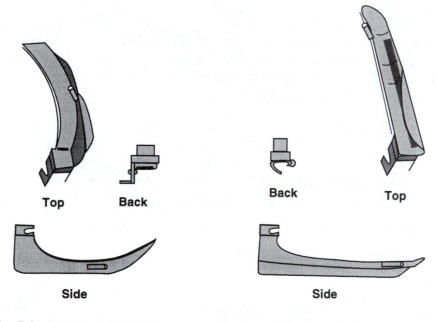

Top   **Back**   **Back**   **Top**

Side   **Side**

Fig. 5-2. Macintosh Blade. Notice the position of the light bulb, the broad, flat blade width, the tall flange for positioning the tongue, and the overall curved shape.

Fig. 5-3. Miller Blade. Notice the position of light bulb, the narrow blade width, the curved channel in center, and the overall

occur in either the cuff or in the balloon assembly. By keeping the tube inside the sterile wrapper you can squeeze the cuff without contaminating it.

You should be aware that endotracheal tube cuffs may break during intubation if they snag on the teeth, etc. Hence tubes, which initially tested fine, may leak after the intubation.

I recommend discarding any tube which leaks. However, there are times when changing a leaking tube in an intubated patient may be difficult. For example, a cuff leak which develops in the middle of head and neck surgery can be hard to treat. You lack easy access to the patient's airway. A long term ventilator patient in the intensive care unit is another example. Occasionally these patients won't tolerate even limited interruption in ventilation without becoming cyanotic. Change the tube if you can.

If you can't, first check the pilot tube. Inflate the cuff until the leak stops and keep the pilot balloon sealed with a closed stopcock or syringe. If the cuff retains air with the pilot tube plugged, then the pilot tube is probably leaking. To keep the cuff inflated use a closed stopcock, a syringe with the plunger firmly taped, or a clamp on the pilot tube itself. I usually avoid clamping the pilot tube itself. This permanently seals the balloon and prevents you from adding any more air in the future.

When the cuff itself leaks, you can temporarily pack the posterior pharynx around the tube with gauze. This helps prevent aspiration and plugs the leak. *Always remember to remove the pack* when you remove or change the tube. Packs left in the pharynx cause potentially fatal airway obstruction. Please view these tricks as temporary measures and not long term solutions.

Placing Your Stylet

Placing your stylet inside the tube comes next (Fig. 5-5). You can intubate without a stylet and you should practice doing so. I always use one in

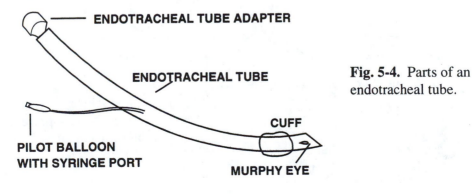

ENDOTRACHEAL TUBE ADAPTER

ENDOTRACHEAL TUBE

PILOT BALLOON WITH SYRINGE PORT

CUFF

MURPHY EYE

Fig. 5-4. Parts of an endotracheal tube.

emergency situations. Failure to intubate rapidly here can lead to aspiration and lack of oxygen. Lubricate the stylet before you insert it. You can use a local anesthetic or lubricating gel, or plain water. Slide the stylet into the tube. Make sure that the stylet does not extend beyond the tip of the tube because the stylet can gouge the trachea in this position. Bend the tip of the endotracheal tube slightly so the tube looks like a hockey stick. This helps you if the patient has an anterior larynx. Make sure that you can still pull the bent stylet out easily. Lubricating gel can occasionally dry out and get sticky. If the stylet has been in the tube a while make sure it's not stuck before you intubate. Nothing is more embarrassing than successfully intubating a patient only to be unable to take the stylet out of the tube.

Final Details

Finally, check that you have suction ready. Also make sure you have the connecting tubing, suction catheters, extension cords, and the power to go with it.

Have the means to ventilate the patient present. Appropriately sized masks, oral and nasal airways (Fig. 5-6), and oxygen should be available. Magill forceps are often useful if you need to do a nasal intubation.

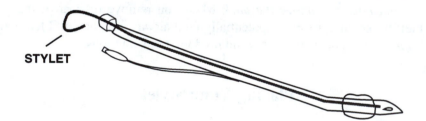

STYLET

Fig. 5-5. Stylet bent like a hockey stick, tip does not extend beyond tube.

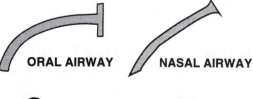

ORAL AIRWAY   **NASAL AIRWAY**

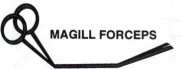

MAGILL FORCEPS

Fig. 5-6. Airway equipment to have present during an intubation.

What To Do When
You Don't Have Optimal Equipment

The reason I originally referred to the list of suggested equipment as optimal is simple. On occasion you may have to intubate a patient without all of the equipment available. Be flexible and let your knowledge of the anatomy and of what you need to accomplish be your guide.

You can intubate a patient without a functioning laryngoscope in several ways. First, use your unlighted laryngoscope or some other similarly shaped instrument such as a bent spoon or oral speculum to lift the jaw. Have an assistant hold a flashlight up to the outside of the larynx. This illuminates the larynx through the skin and the vocal cords light up. Once you can see them you can pass your tube. You can also intubate by feel. Place the fingers of your left hand inside the patient's mouth until your index and middle fingers straddle the larynx. Pass the endotracheal tube with your right hand, using your left hand to direct it between the vocal cords.

If you don't have a ventilation bag use mouth-to-mouth or mouth-to-tube ventilation.

Active suction is wonderful. Improvise it if you don't have it. Quickly turn the patient on his or her side to clear the airway with gauze or other tissue. Use a syringe bulb or a syringe attached to some IV extension tubing.

Have someone place an ear to the chest and listen for breath sounds if you don't have a stethoscope.

Always open your mind to alternatives. Flexibility saves patient's lives.

6 ORAL INTUBATION OF THE ADULT PATIENT

Many of you have already intubated an intubation mannequin and therefore are familiar with the basic technique. However, intubating the dummy differs from intubating the typical patient. You should recognize these differences before you approach your first patient.

The Dummy vs. the Real Thing

The dummy's plastic face is very stiff and noncompliant. You've probably noticed that the mouth already lies fully open and is difficult to open further. In contrast, you must open the patient's mouth, and do so without getting in the way of your laryngoscope. Being soft and very compliant, the human cheek will hang limply, obstructing the view.

The dummy's head is so light that it takes little effort to lift the entire mannequin off the table. Often instructors have to hold the mannequin on the table to help the trainee out. In contrast, the average adult head weighs about 5 lbs. The added weight makes balancing the head on the blade and lifting the head into the proper alignment technically more difficult. Holding the head in proper position, especially through a long and difficult intubation, is very tiring.

You can often see the dummy's larynx even without the laryngoscope lit because the pale plastic reflects light so well. This isn't the case in humans. The mucous membranes are dark. The larynx, deep in the hole, lies in shadow. Placing the laryngoscope light correctly and then interpreting the view is easier if you know what the real larynx looks like.

The dummy's tongue is fairly firm, difficult to shift from side to side. However, it will remain out of the way of your blade. Your patient's tongue will be a soft, very slippery mound of flesh. It will invariably be in the worst position to block your view if you fail to control it.

Psychology is the final difference. You know that you cannot hurt the dummy even if you fail completely. Every beginner fears his or her first patient intubation. Even if you can intubate the dummy with your eyes closed I guarantee that your first few intubations will be frightening. This is normal. You worry about failure because you doubt your ability to succeed. You are fearful of what will happen if you fail. However, if you approach the patient with gentle, purposeful movements, and ventilate the patient between attempts, your likelihood of hurting the patient is low. Panic hurts patients. Apprehension does not. Use your apprehension as a tool to heighten your awareness and to promote caution. If you believe you can intubate, you will.

Intubating the Adult

To orally intubate you need to bring the path from the incisor teeth to the larynx into a straight line. This path has three axes (Fig. 6-1):

1. axis of the cavity of the mouth (oral axis)
2. axis of the cavity of the pharynx (pharyngeal axis)
3. axis of the larynx and trachea (laryngeal axis)

The angle of the axis of the mouth to the larynx is 90°. That of the pharynx to the trachea is obtuse. Aligning them is merely a matter of applied mechanics. You make this alignment by moving the patient's head and neck and then using the laryngoscope blade to make the final adjustment. Other techniques can be

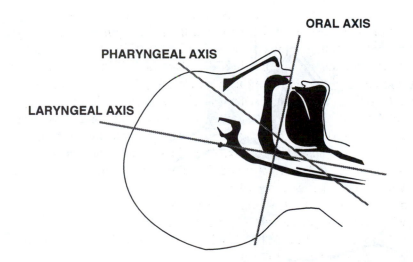

Fig. 6-1. The three axes with the head in neutral position.

used if you shouldn't move the patient's head, such as in cervical trauma and some facial fractures. We'll discuss these situations in Chapter 12. Here we discuss the basic intubation technique assuming optimal conditions.

Place the patient's head at the level of your xyphoid, the lower tip of your breast bone for the best mechanical advantage. You can, however, intubate in any position.

The act of intubation alternates hands. One hand positions the patient for the next action by the other hand. With practice, coordinating the alternating hand movements becomes natural.

Raise the patient's head about 10 cm (4 inches) off the bed by placing a folded sheet or other object under their head. Leave the shoulders on the bed (Fig. 6-2). This aligns the pharyngeal and laryngeal axes. The cervical spine is now straight and the patient is in the so-called "sniffing position." Picture how someone out of breath holds her head: forward and tilted slightly back. We automatically straighten the airway to minimize resistance when we want to move a lot of air easily.

Tilt the head into extension with your right hand. This brings all the axes into alignment (Fig. 6-3). Hold it there momentarily either by using your upper chest or your left hand to anchor it (Fig. 6-4a, b). Don't stick your fingers into the patient's eyes as you do this! Anchoring the head frees your right hand. Open the mouth with your right hand by placing your thumb on the lower jaw and your middle finger on the upper jaw (Fig. 6-5). The position is similar to snapping your fingers. By using a pushing rather than a spreading motion, you can open

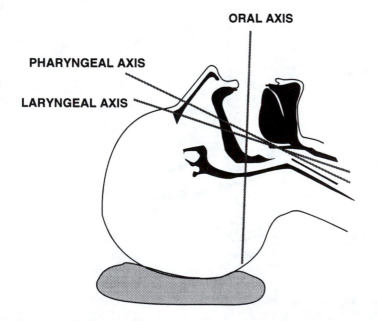

ORAL AXIS

PHARYNGEAL AXIS

LARYNGEAL AXIS

Fig. 6-2. The three axes with the head in the "sniffing" position.

the mouth wider and more forcefully. Make sure that you place your fingers as far to the right side of the mouth as you can. This keeps your fingers out of the way of the blade.

Your right hand now does double duty. It holds the mouth open as wide as it can. By pulling toward you it also holds the head in extension. You can now step back from the head and use your left hand to pick up and insert the blade (Fig. 6-6).

Insertion of the blade should be delicate and deliberate. Hold the handle in your left hand, blade down, pointing away from you (Fig. 6-7). Don't clench your fist because this decreases control and causes early fatigue. Because my hands are small, I place my hand lower down on the handle. I rest my fifth finger on the blade and wrap my hand around the handle. This puts the heel of my hand on the junction between blade and handle and allows me to fine tune the angle of the blade. Notice how easily you can change the angle of the blade by tilting your wrist (Fig. 6-7).

With the mouth open, insert the blade between the teeth, slightly to the right of the tongue (Fig. 6-8a, b). Don't push on the teeth as you do so. Also avoid catching the lips between the blade and the teeth. I use my right index finger to sweep the lips out of the way of the blade as I insert it.

Slowly advance the blade with your left hand until you see the tip of the epiglottis, your first important landmark. Simultaneously sweep the tongue to the

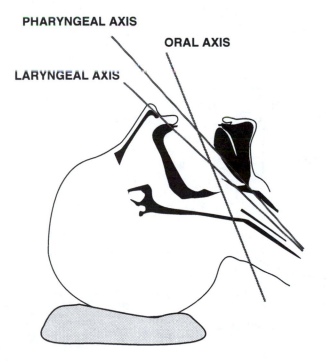

PHARYNGEAL AXIS

ORAL AXIS

LARYNGEAL AXIS

Fig. 6-3. The three axes after extending the head.

left as you advance (Fig. 6-9a, b). This leaves your blade in the midline of the mouth with the tongue pushed out of the way. When you lift the jaw upward you have an unobstructed view of the larynx (Fig. 6-10a, b, c). Pressure from the tip of a curved blade in the vallecula pulls the epiglottis forward. Placement of the blade is critical. If you place the blade in the center of the tongue it will mound up and you will see nothing. You must sweep the tongue to the left or you will see nothing.

a.

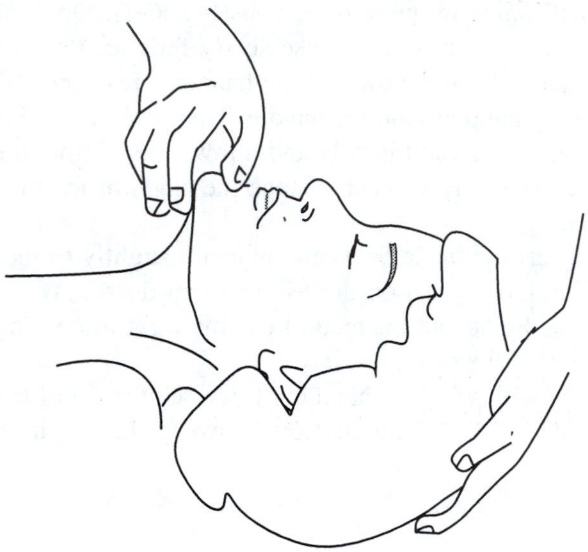

b.

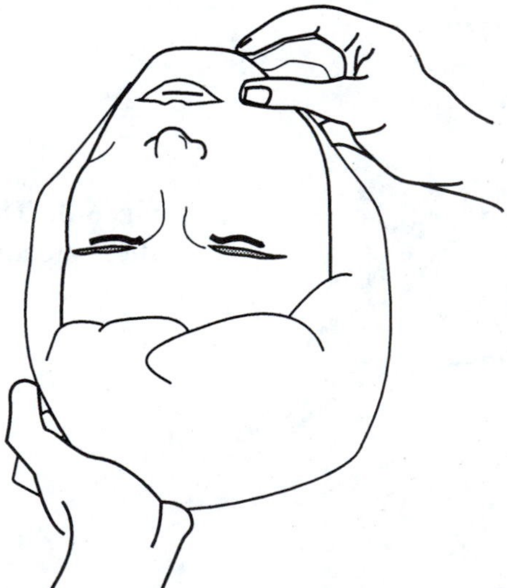

Fig. 6-4 a, b. Tilt the head back, place in the sniffing position.

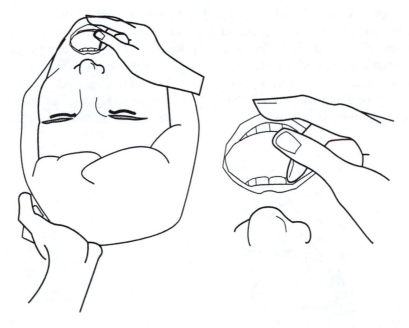

Fig. 6-5. Open the mouth with your right hand, your fingers as far to the right of the mouth as possible. Notice the positioning of the fingers.

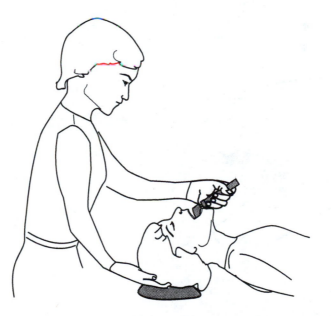

Fig. 6-6. Keep your back and your left arm straight to optimize mechanical advantage.

For optimal mechanical advantage lift upward with the left arm held fairly straight. Lift on a line connecting the patient's head with the intersection of the opposite ceiling and the wall (Fig. 6-11). Keeping your arm straight gives you the strength of your shoulders to lift the head. It prevents you from using the teeth as a fulcrum — dangerous for the teeth. And it allows you to use binocular vision for depth perception. The typical beginners (Fig. 6-12) hunch close to the patient, bend the elbow completely, and place the right eye practically into

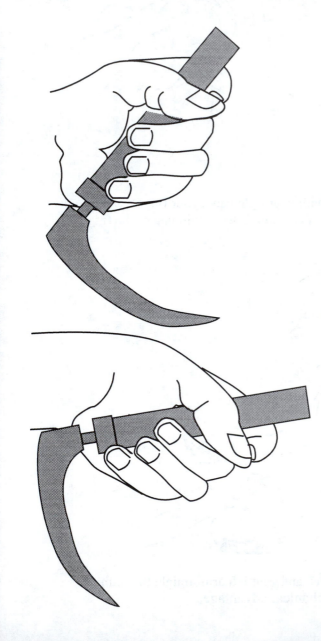

Fig. 6-7. You can easily change the angle of the blade by rotating your wrist.

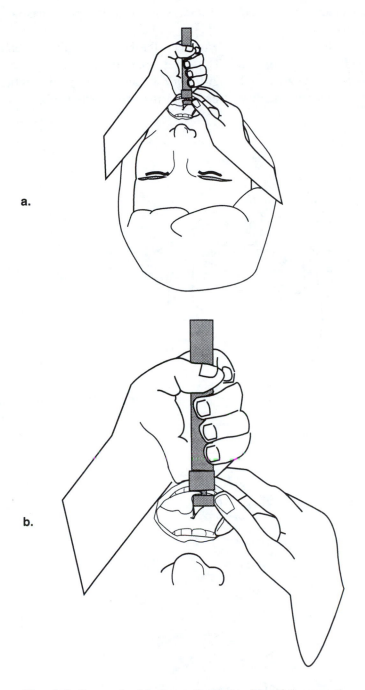

a.

b.

Fig. 6-8. Insert the blade on the right side of the mouth,
not in the middle of the tongue.

the patient's mouth. They then can't understand why he or she has no leverage or control. Don't do this.

Back to the intubation. We left you with the head virtually suspended from the blade held in your left hand. This frees your right hand to place the tube. Use a 7.0-8.5 for a woman and a 7.5-9.0 for a man. The larger the tube, the less resistence to breathing there will be. Hold the pre-selected tube in your right

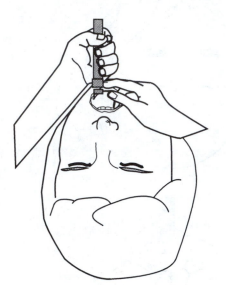

a.

b.

Fig. 6-9. Slide the blade to the left, pushing the tongue out of the way. Lift upward on the lower jaw.

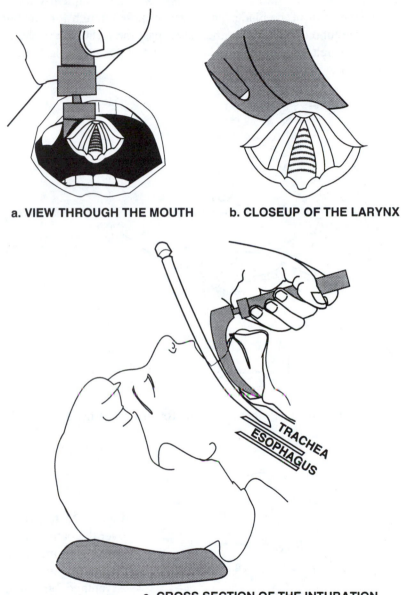

a. VIEW THROUGH THE MOUTH   **b. CLOSEUP OF THE LARYNX**

TRACHEA
ESOPHAGUS

c. CROSS SECTION OF THE INTUBATION

Fig. 6-10. Visualization of the cords and passing the endotracheal tube.

hand like a pencil, curve forward. In one smooth motion pass the tube into the
larynx through the cords (Fig. 6-13). If the patient is breathing, time the forward thrust for inspiration when the cords open. During expiration, the tube
may bounce off the cords into the esophagus. Beginners frequently try to pass
the tube down the slot in the blade. The slot is not big enough for this purpose.
Instead, pass the tube to the right of the blade, past the right side of the tongue.
This is the major reason why the blade has to be as far to the left side of the
mouth as possible.

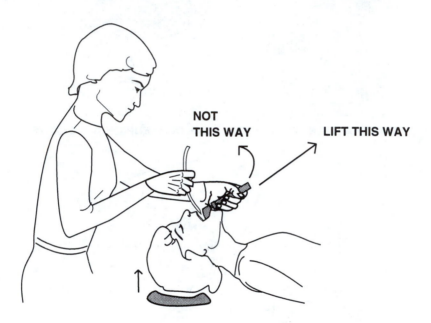

Fig. 6-11. Proper technique for lifting the head.

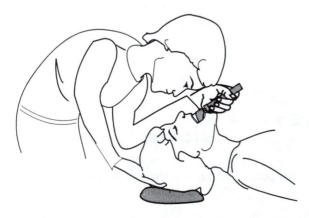

Fig. 6-12. Avoid stooping
over the patient and
bending your arm. You
lose mechanical
advantage, binocular
vision, and

Try to watch the tube pass through the cords into the trachea. Although there may be a blind spot impairing your view at the moment of intubation, you can often see the arytenoids behind the tube after proper placement. Don't relax and pull the blade out without trying to be sure of success with your own eyes. Get into the habit of seeing the tube between the cords and you will be less likely to intubate the esophagus.

Stop advancing the tube when you see the cuff completely pass the cords. Carefully hold the tube where it exits the right side of the mouth and remove the blade with your left hand. To inflate the cuff to the minimal sealing pressure, apply constant airway pressure of about 20 mmHg. Then fill the cuff with air until the tracheal leak just disappears. Excessive cuff inflation can damage mucosa by impairing its blood supply.

Before doing anything else, be sure that the tube is in the trachea. Listen for the presence and equality of breath sounds over both lung fields and for the absence of gurgling sounds over the stomach. Never assume that the tube is in the trachea until you have checked it yourself. More details on this later.

Securing the Tube

Next, tape the tube securely. Only your taping stands between the patient and extubation. To start, notice the depth of the tube by looking at the numbers. Remember which number lines up with the front gum line: typically 21 cm for a

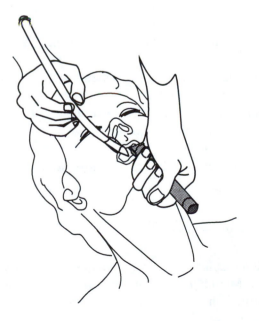

Fig. 6-13. Another view of passing the tube into the larynx.

woman, 22 cm for a man. For a child the depth in centimeters should equal the age in years divided by 2 plus 12. For example a four year old child should have the tube inserted to a depth of 14cm (or 4 divided by 2 plus 12). Tape the tube to the side of the mouth. It usually doesn't matter on which side of the mouth you tape the tube. Most of us tape it on the right side since the tube already exits from that side. There are many acceptable ways of taping the tube. Figures 6-14 and 6-15 show two ways. These methods have several factors in common. First, having the tube in the exact corner of the mouth is more comfortable for the patient. It avoids the patient pushing the tube out with the tongue. It also makes it easier for others to suction the mouth and place oral airways if needed. Second, you don't leave a tape tether. Tape extensions let the tube slide in or out of the mouth, risking either mainstem intubation or extubation. Finally, you avoid taping over the vermillion border or edge of the lip. You can tear this border when you remove the tape, especially in babies and geriatric patients. In addition, tape over the lips gets wet from saliva and loses its grip.

Once the tube is taped, check again that the tube still lies in the trachea.

If you need the tube on the left side of the mouth, then you will have to move the tube. Hold the tube securely with your right hand where it exits the mouth and rest your hand on the cheek (Fig. 6-16). Holding further out on the tube is unstable and risks extubation if the head moves. Take a tongue blade, or your laryngoscope blade, with your left hand and open the mouth. Push the tongue firmly down. Under direct vision move the tube from the groove on the right side of the tongue to the groove on the left. Don't let the tube overlie the tongue as this allows the patient to "tongue" it out. Hold the tube securely with either hand and immediately check that the tube is still in the trachea. **I can't emphasize strongly enough that you must verify good breath sounds bilaterally anytime the tube or the patient moves**. Extubation and mainstem intubation can occur at any time.

Tape sticks poorly to hair. Taping endotracheal tubes in patients with beards and mustaches requires an alteration in technique. One can use the above methods after applying benzoin to the hair. A more secure method uses an "around the neck" tape as in Fig. 6-17. You can use this method whenever you need greater tube stabilization, for example, during prone positioning or transportation. Don't tape too tightly because your tape might constrict the neck like a tourniquet and cause facial swelling.

Straight vs. Curved Blades

The straight blade, such as the Miller, actually picks up the epiglottis during the intubation. The curved MacIntosh (Mac) blade fits into the vallecula, the dip between the tongue and the epiglottis. While the technique is the same, the

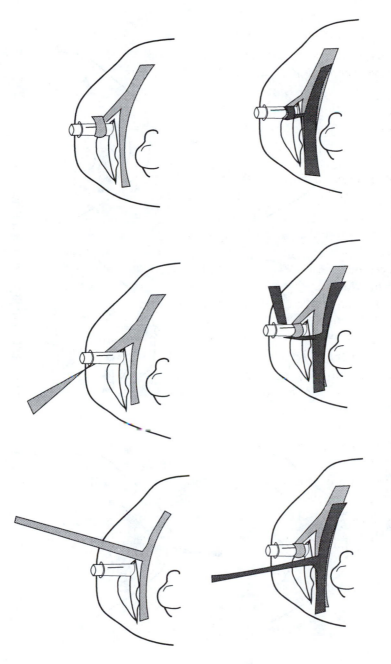

Fig. 6-14. One method to tape an endotracheal tube. See text for description.

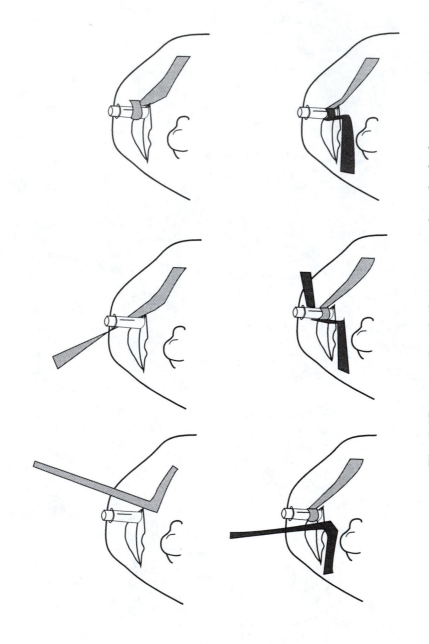

Fig. 6-15. A second method to tape an endotracheal tube.

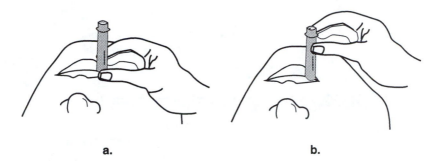

a.   b.

Fig. 6-16. When holding an endotracheal tube hold it where it exits the mouth as in **a**. Rest your hand against the cheek so that you move as the head moves. Exutbation is more likely if you hold the tube as in **b.**

effect on the tissues differs between the blades. The curved blade lifts the epiglottis passively by pulling the tissue folds attached at its base. The straight blade flattens the tongue and actively lifts the epiglottis. See Figures 6-18, 6-19, 6-20 for illustrations of these effects.

You can begin to see that a straight blade might be more helpful in situations where there is little room to displace the tongue and attached tissues forward. Patients with short necks, high larynxes, or obesity frequently need straight blades. Straight blades can also work better in patients with larynxes fixed from scar, trauma, or mass effect. Again, displacement is not as critical. Remember that you can pick up the epiglottis with the Mac or use the Miller in the vallecula if the need arises.

In the average patient, it really doesn't matter which blade you use. Many beginners find the Mac blade easier to use. It's larger flange holds the tongue off to the left and makes it easier to balance the head. It is more forgiving of placement errors. Straight blades often give you a better view but are harder to use. Practice with both blades on the easy patients. That way, when a difficult intubation comes along you control the anatomy rather than letting the anatomy dictate to you. We'll discuss more on these situations later. Look at the pictures and get a feel for how your blade moves the tissues around.

Further Reading

Mallampati SR, Gratt SP, Gugino LD, Desai SP, et. al.: A clinical sign to predict difficult tracheal intubation: a prospective study. *Can. Anaesth. Soc. J.* 1985; 32: 4: 429

Stoelting RK, Miller RD: Airway Management. *Basics of Anesthesia.* Edited by Stoelting RK, Miller RD. New York. Churchill-Livingstone 1984, 153-165

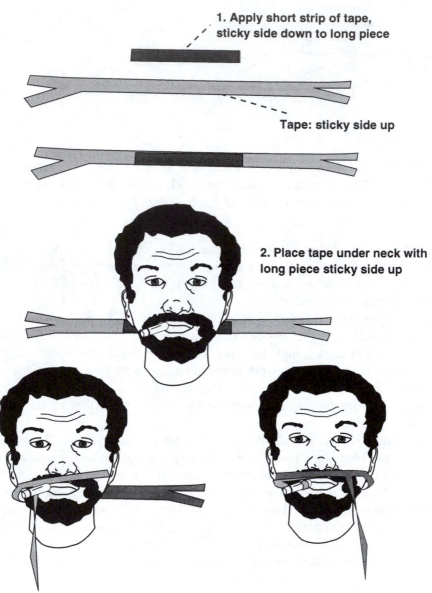

Fig. 6-17. Taping an endotracheal tube in a bearded patient.

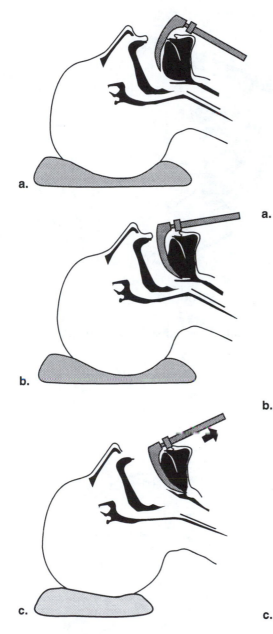

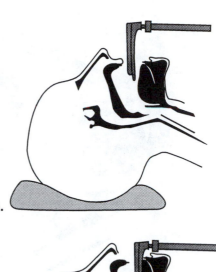

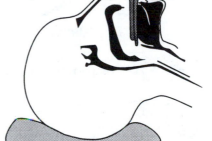

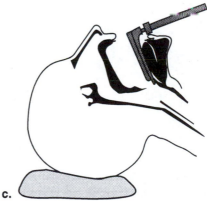

Fig. 6-18. Placement of a curved blade. Notice the position of the tip in the vallecula.

Fig. 6-19. Placement of a straight blade. Note that the blade flattens the tissue. The tip is on the epiglotis.

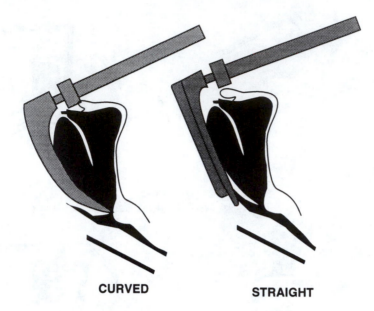

CURVED   **STRAIGHT**

Fig. 6-20. Comparison of the placement of curved and straight blades.

7 COMMON ERRORS AND HOW TO AVOID THEM

Inexperienced intubators often make several fairly common errors. Every year new trainees repeat them.

Positioning Errors

Poor head placement is the most common error. Sometimes you can't avoid it, such as during a cardiac arrest with the patient on the floor. Frequently you can optimize position with pillows. Having an assistant stabilize or lift the head, or changing the bed height, are also helpful. These changes are fast, easy to perform, and often forgotten in the heat of battle. They make the intubation easier and therefore less stressful and more likely to succeed.

Keep your left arm and back as straight as possible. Hunching over the patient, a common mistake, makes intubation more difficult because it impairs your mechanical advantage (Fig. 7-1).

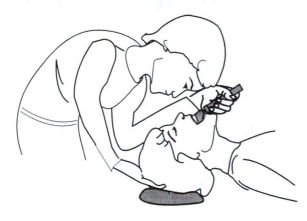

Fig. 7-1. Don't hunch over the patient. Keep your back and left arm as straight as possible.

In the rush to extend the patient's head the intubator will frequently place fingers in the patient's eyes (Fig. 7-2). After all, the orbital ridge is a convenient place to grab and pull. In their preoccupation, they sometimes don't notice themselves doing this.

When opening the mouth, inexperienced fingers grab the middle teeth. This never leaves enough room to pass the blade into the mouth. Place your fingers on the far right. Use the finger positioning shown in Fig. 7-3 and use a pushing rather than a spreading motion.

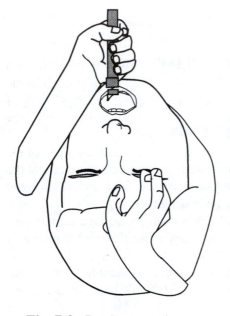

Fig. 7-2. Don't gouge the eyes.

Left-handed Intubation

Open the mouth as widely as you can. You are far less likely to damage teeth or gums if you give yourself room to maneuver and see.

Most people are right handed. Therefore, many people instinctively reach for the laryngoscope with their right hand. They discover their mistake when they find themselves with their right hand blocking their view and with no way for their left hand to pass a tube over their right. Standard laryngoscopes are held in the non-dominant left hand because this hand merely provides a stable platform. The dominant right hand needs all the coordination and dexterity to manipulate the tube. Unfortunately, this leaves left

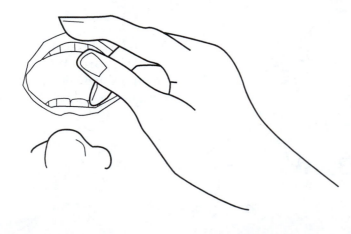

Fig. 7-3. Finger position for opening the mouth.

handed intubators in an awkward position. As just pointed out, the standard blades are held in the left hand. Reversing them doesn't work. Although the southpaw can purchase a left handed blade, which is a mirror image of the standard blade, I don't recommend this. It is far better for you to train yourself to do it "backwards." Training yourself on left handed tools puts you at a major disadvantage when only right handed tools are available. Most hospitals only stock right handed instruments. It may not be fair, but it's definitely more practical. Most left handed intubators use the standard blade, just like they learned to use right handed scissors and other tools when they were kids. It's just a matter of practice.

Problems with Techniques

As mentioned earlier, a blade placed in the center of the tongue produces a mound of tissue that blocks the view (Fig. 7-4). Make sure that you slide the blade as far to the left side of the mouth as you can. This gets the tongue out of your way. It also places the blade close to the midline, a very stable position for lifting and balancing the head.

Leaving the blade too far to the right often gives you an excellent view of the cords but no room to pass the tube (Fig. 7-5). Sometimes you can't even get the tube into the mouth. This may be your problem if you routinely ask an assistant to pull the right corner of the mouth out of the way.

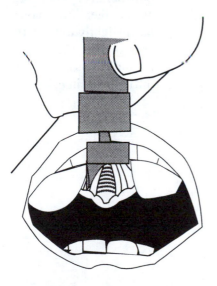

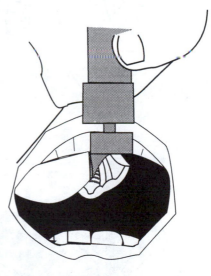

Fig. 7-4. The tongue will get in the way if you place the blade in the middle.

Fig. 7-5. Push the blade as far to the left as possible or there won't be room to pass the tube.

Sometimes you have a great view with a straight blade but can't pass the tube. Straight Miller blades have the light bulb on the right. When this light bulb is angled toward the right it often deflects the endotracheal tube. If you simply rotate the blade slightly to the left, you will raise the bulb out of the way (Fig. 7-6).

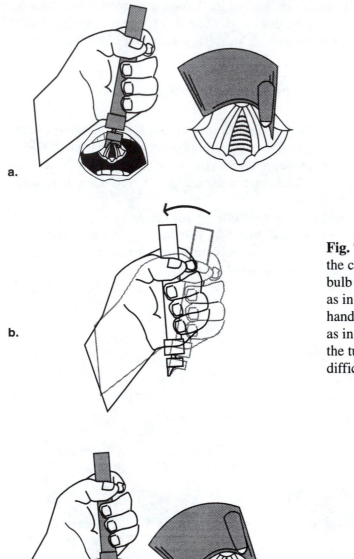

Fig. 7-6. If you can see the cords, but the light bulb deflects your tube, as in **a**, then rotate your hand slightly to the left as in **b.** This often allows the tube to pass without difficulty as in **c**.

The other common error with a straight blade is inserting it too deep, into the esophagus. If you can't identify any landmarks, slowly pull the blade back. Often the larynx will fall into view. A straight blade can "tent" the esophagus and make it look like vocal cords if you haven't actually seen both.

Failure to lift the lower jaw upward is another common error. Inexperienced intubators place their blade very gently, and then barely lift the jaw. They fear hurting the patient. They don't realize that unless they lift the epiglottis and tongue up, they will see nothing. This leads to the next error. Failing to see anything, they then use the blade like a lever to lift the epiglottis. The only fulcrum available is the front row of teeth (Fig. 7-7). This is very dangerous for the teeth. Never lever on the teeth. Always lift. Properly done, you will actually lift the head off the bed. This won't hurt the patient.

Edentulous or partially edentulous people frequently fool the intubator into thinking he or she has lifted enough. Without teeth you see a great view of the larynx without lifting the jaw. Without the lift, however, the mouth is barely wide enough to pass the tube (Fig. 7-8). Always remember to lift.

Once you have an understanding of the intubation procedure and the purpose of each step, you can easily avoid the common errors.

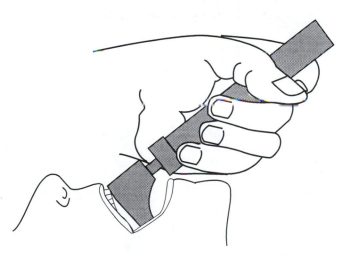

Fig. 7-7. Don't push on the teeth. Lift upward instead. Like tennis: keep the wrist stiff and the elbow straight.

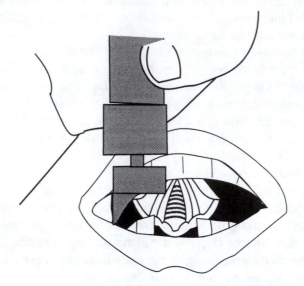

Fig. 7-8. You can see the larynx because the
teeth are missing, even though the mouth is
not wide enough to pass the tube.

8 TESTS FOR TUBE PLACEMENT

After intubation, check immediately that the tube is positioned correctly in the trachea and not in the esophagus or mainstem bronchus (Fig. 8-1, 8-2). Even expert intubators occasionally intubate the esophagus. This is not a problem as long as you recognize the error and correct it at once.

Seven Steps for Correct Tube Placement

One of the first ways to be sure of tube placement is to see the endotracheal tube between the vocal cords. As you start to remove your laryngoscope blade

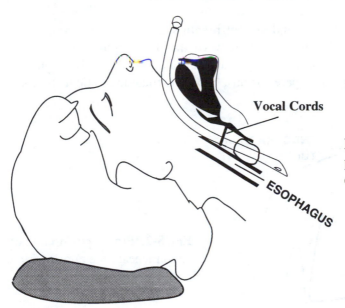

Vocal Cords

ESOPHAGUS

Fig. 8-1. Correct position of the endotracheal tube.

look for the cords. Remove the blade slowly. Carefully hold the endotracheal tube to avoid pulling the tube out with the blade. Now perform the following tests.

1. Listen over both sides of the chest for the presence of breath sounds. A tube placed too far down the trachea will lie in one mainstem bronchus and block the other. In this case you will hear breath sounds only on one side of the chest.

2. Listen over the stomach with a stethoscope for a gurgling sound when you ventilate with your bag. This indicates an esophageal intubation.

3. Look for condensation forming inside the tube with each breath. This indicates tracheal placement.

4. Watch for the chest to rise each time you give a breath.

5. If the patient is awake and the cuff is up, he or she will no longer be able to speak.

6. If breathing spontaneously, you will feel air movement with your hand placed over the tube.

7. If you have an end-tidal CO_2 apparatus, attach it and turn it on. CO_2 won't be present with an esophageal intubation.

Esophageal Intubations

Gurgling over the stomach and lack of breath sounds over the chest means the tube is in the esophagus. Calmly remove the tube, having your suction ready. Removal of a tube from the esophagus can cause either passive regurgitation or active vomiting so prepare for this. Next, ventilate the patient by mask

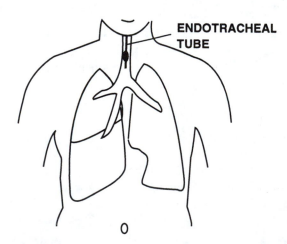

ENDOTRACHEAL TUBE

Fig. 8-2. Proper positioning of endotracheal tube above carina.

until you are feel that the patient is adequately oxygenated. The color of the lips, nail beds, and conjunctivae of the eyes are pink if the patient is oxygenated. Try again. I tell a helper, if I have one, to provide cricoid pressure after removing the tube. The risk of passive regurgitation is higher due to the increased volume of air now in the stomach. Also the passage of the tube into the esophagus opens the sphincters and may decrease their tone. I maintain cricoid pressure until after I place the final tube in the trachea.

Usually there's no doubt about whether the tube lies in the trachea or the esophagus. Unfortunately, there are rare instances when you can't easily tell. It's important to know that you can occasionally hear breath sounds over the chest with an esophageal intubation. These breath sounds, however, will be extremely faint and muffled. The chest will rise poorly. Lung compliance, or the ease of inflating the lungs, will be extremely poor. Condensation does not form inside the tube with each breath. It will be hard to keep your bag filled with gas.

The absence of gurgles over the stomach is not fail-safe. I have seen one case where the stomach was distended with air. The tube cuff effectively sealed the esophagus and there were no audible gurgles over the stomach. We heard faint breath sounds and we were easily able to keep the bag filled with gas because the esophagus was sealed. We suspected esophageal placement because the compliance was extremely poor. Checking the position of the tube with a laryngoscope notified us of its misplacement before injury to the patient occured.

In comparison, patients with severe bronchospasm start with extremely faint breath sounds and very stiff lung compliance. Their chest barely rises. The endotracheal tube may be correctly placed but you sometimes can't tell by listening to the chest alone. Children, on the other hand, have breath sounds that on occasion seem audible over the big toe. You might hear faint "breath" sounds in children with an esophageal intubation.

These real life situations make detection of esophageal intubations more difficult. If you have any doubts about the correct placement of your endotracheal tube *don't hesitate to look with your laryngoscope.*

Having and using an end-tidal CO_2 measuring apparatus will detect all esophageal intubations. The presence of CO_2 in the exhalate can only mean placement of the tube in the trachea. If you are fortunate enough to have such a machine available, you should learn to use it.

Mainstem Intubation

A mainstem intubation occurs when the endotracheal tube extends down one mainstem bronchus, ventilating one lung but obstructing the other (Fig. 8-3). Usually the tube advances down the right side because the right mainstem bronchus is straighter. Louder breath sounds on one side of the chest may mean a mainstem intubation. To cure a mainstem intubation, pull the tube back until you hear breath sounds on both sides of the chest. Secure the tube to prevent it from sliding back down the trachea.

One word of caution. Before you reposition the tube look at the numbers and see if the depth of insertion is correct for that particular patient. This depth is about 21 cm at the teeth in a woman, 22 cm in a man. For a child, determine the depth in cm by dividing the age in years by 2 and then adding 12. If the depth seems correct ask yourself whether another reason for unequal breath sounds exists. Pneumothorax, pneumonectomy, or pleural effusion also cause unequal breath sounds. If the answer is no, then slowly back the tube out until you hear equal breath sounds. However, if the breath sounds do not become equal as the tube gets shallower, stop. Recheck the depth of tube placement by laryngoscopy (to ensure the cuff is below the cords), get an X-ray, and look for other reasons for inequality.

Tube Is Too Shallow

Sometimes after inflating your tube cuff you'll notice a persistent leak. Adding more air to the cuff might make the leak worse. There are two possibilities. The first is that the cuff has a hole in it or that the pilot balloon leaks. In both of these situations the pilot balloon is soft when you squeeze it. The second possibility is that the cuff is above the vocal cords (Fig. 8-4). You can ventilate the patient because the tube tip lies in the trachea, but the cuff can't totally seal the leak. Suspect a cuff above the cords if you can't get rid of a leak, the

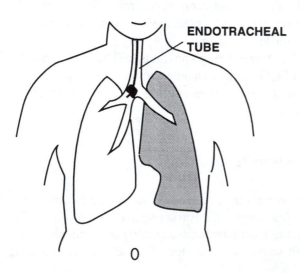

ENDOTRACHEAL TUBE

Fig. 8-3. Right mainstem intubation shaded lung not ventilated.

pilot balloon is tense, and the tube is shallow. Repeat laryngoscopy can differentiate the two.

Further Reading

Pollard BJ, James B: Accidental intubation of the esophagus. *Anaes. Intens. Care* 1980; 8: 183

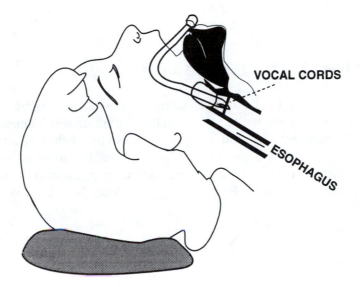

VOCAL CORDS

ESOPHAGUS

Fig. 8-4. Tube bowed in the posterior pharynx, cuff is above the cords.

9 VENTILATING AND INTUBATING THE CHILD

Children Are Not Small Adults

Pediatric physiology and airway anatomy differ in many ways from the adult, differences you must recognize to successfully ventilate and intubate children. Compare the anatomy of a child in Figures 9-1 and 9-2 with the anatomy of an adult in Figures 1-1 and 1-2 (pp. 13). Table 9-1 summarizes these differences.

Airway management is critical. Children develop hypoxemia faster than adults because their smaller lungs and higher metabolic rates give them less

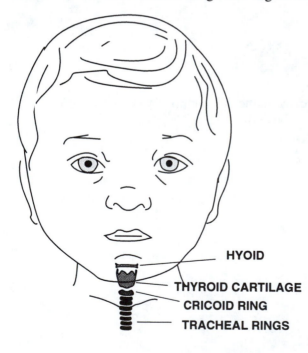

Fig. 9-1. Notice how much higher in the neck the larynx lies in the infant.

HYOID

THYROID CARTILAGE

CRICOID RING

TRACHEAL RINGS

Table 9-1. Comparing Infant and Adult Airways.

	Infant	Adult
Tongue	relatively larger	relatively smaller
Larynx	opposite 2nd and 3rd cervical vertebrae	opposite 4th, 5th, and 6th cervical vertebrae
Epiglottis	"U" shaped, short, stiff	flat, flexible, erect
Hyoid/Thyroid separation	very close	further apart
Glottis	1/2 cartilage	1/4 cartilage
Arytenoids	inclined inferiorly	horizontal
Vocal Cords	concave	horizontal
Cricoid	plate forms funnel	plate vertical
Smallest Diameter	cricoid ring	vocal cord aperture
Consistency of Cartilage	soft	firm
Shape of Head	pronounced occiput	flatter occiput

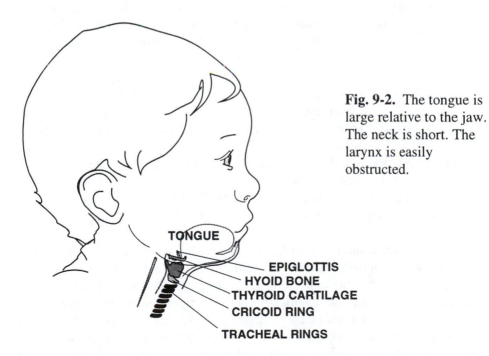

Fig. 9-2. The tongue is large relative to the jaw. The neck is short. The larynx is easily obstructed.

TONGUE

EPIGLOTTIS
HYOID BONE
THYROID CARTILAGE
CRICOID RING

TRACHEAL RINGS

oxygen reserve. The immature lungs of infants are not as efficient, and their poorly developed muscles of respiration tire easily. In addition, infants and young children are often anemic, giving them less hemoglobin in their blood to carry oxygen.

Hypoxic adults remain tachycardic for a long time before this compensatory mechanism fails and bradycardia begins. Unlike adults, children develop brady-cardia as soon as hypoxia starts because of their immature nervous system. A slow heart rate delivers even less oxygen. You must recognize and correct hy-poxia very quickly or cardiac arrest may occur.

Pediatric airway management is similar to the adult with several important differences. The large occiput flexes the head forward when lying supine, col-lapsing the tongue and soft tissues over the larynx and causing airway obstruc-tion. Tilting the head into extension opens the airway. However, extreme extension or flexion of the child's head can compress the trachea because the cartilage is soft, impairing ventilation. A more neutral, slightly extended posi-tion is best.

Placing a small folded towel under an infant's shoulders sometimes helps to open the airway. Pillows are seldom needed and may worsen obstruction. Lifting the jaw further opens the airway. Keep your fingers on the boney mandi-ble. Pressure on the soft tissue under the chin may actually increase obstruction. Press gently if you need cricoid pressure.

You may need an oral airway to adequately ventilate these children. The ton-sillar and adenoidal tissue fills the "dead space" in the nose and posterior phar-ynx and can cause partial obstruction. Oral airways used in conscious or semi-conscious patients risk vomiting, aspiration, and issue damage. If placed incor-rectly, oral airway can increase airway obstruction by pushing the tongue back.

Nasal airways can cause nose-bleeds in children with hypertrophied ade-noids. I only use them in these children as a last resort. Lubricate the nasal air-way well before insertion and be gentle as you pass it. Adenoidal tissue can plug nasal airways, as well as nasal endotracheal tubes, after passing through the nose. This creates the risk of obstruction or of aspiration of tissue. Pass a suction catheter through the tube while the tip still lies in the posterior pharynx to clear it before pushing it further into the trachea.

Another way to establish an airway is to hold the mouth open under the mask. I use the hand grip shown in Fig. 9-3 a, b. This mimics the action of an oral airway.

Children differ from infants in having teeth, often in various stages of attach-ment. If you have the time, always look for loose or missing teeth before you start.

The vocal cords in the child have a concave upward shape, rather than the horizontal shape of the adult. While this doesn't affect our ability to intubate the child, it can affect our ability to ventilate him. We often use positive pressure with bag and mask to treat partial airway obstruction or laryngospasm. This works because the positive pressure pushes the vocal cords downward and slightly apart. Once the cords separate even a little bit, the positive pressure expands the space below them. This forces the arytenoids apart, opening the airway. Horizontal cords should separate more easily under positive pressure than concave cords, which might overlap more forcefully. To break laryngospasm in a child, we combine positive pressure with chin thrust. Thrusting the chin forward puts tension on the arytenoids, and pulls them apart. The gap produced allows pressurization of the space below and the spasm usually breaks.

The inflating pressures needed to ventilate an infant or child are much less than for an adult. Use smaller breathes to avoid barotrauma, pneumothorax, and stomach distension. Stomach distension causes vomiting and prevents full lung expansion, causing hypoxemia.

Both children and adults have a normal tidal volume of about 7 cc per kg of body weight. A 70 kg adult has a tidal volume of 500 cc. A 10 kg child has a 70 cc tidal volume. use a bag appropriate for the size of the tidal volume if possible. You can better judge both the pressure and the volume delivered by using a half to one liter bag instead of an adult bag. When in doubt, have an assistant listen to breathe sounds to confirm ventilation.

Children need a higher ventilatory rate than adults because of their faster metabolic rates. Ventilate infants at 35-40, children at 20-30, and teenagers at 10-20 breathes per minute.

Children less than 8 years old have heart rates faster than 100 beats per minute. If a child develops bradycardia while you are ventilating him assume that the cause is hypoxia. Recheck your hand position and oxygen source. Be certain you are ventilating. Increase the depth and rate of ventilation along with the inspired oxygen concentration. The heart rate usually returns to normal quickly although atropine may also be needed.

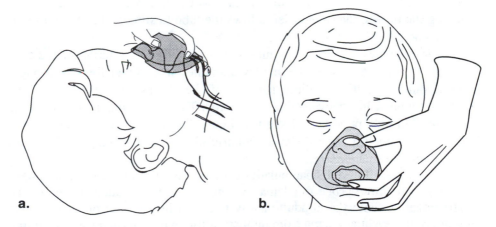

a.   **b.**

Fig. 9-3a, b. Technique to hold the mouth open under the mask. Pull lower jaw upward and toward the feet by hooking the lower fingers under the mandible. Maintain the seal with your thumb and index finger.

Mechanical advantage explains why these differences force us to alter our intubation technique. Note that infants differ the most from the adult and that these differences slowly diminish as the child ages. In other words, the older the child, the more like an adult he or she becomes for intubation.

First, everything in the pediatric airway is smaller, making manipulations with adult hands and equipment technically more difficult.

Second, the cartilage is very soft and pliable. Cricoid pressure or extremes of head position can cause actual obstruction of the airway.

Children have pronounced occiputs, almost a built-in sniffing position. I rarely use a towel under the head of a child less than 9 years old for intubation. Small infants sometimes have too much "sniffing position." Their heads flex on their necks when laying flat on the table. Placing a small towel under such an infant's back corrects the angle of approach.

A tongue that is larger relative to the size of the mouth gives us less room to work. It is more difficult to sweep the tongue to the left and displace it forward. The smaller separation between the hyoid and the thyroid cartilage also makes displacing the tongue and associated structures forward more difficult. For these reasons we most frequently choose a straight blade for intubating children.

Using a curved blade in the vallecula often folds the epiglottis down over the vocal cords, blocking the view (Fig. 9-4). The higher anatomical position of the larynx in the neck causes this. However, the angles are such that picking up the epiglottis with the straight blade creates a clear passage.

Picking up the epiglottis in a child of less than five years old can be difficult due to its short, stiff, "U" shaped form. Meticulous placement of the tip of the blade is necessary.

The arytenoids in the child incline. Because of this slant, the pediatric tube can hang up on the anterior commissure when passing it into the larynx. Rotating the tube to the right or left allows the tube to slip off the anterior commissure and pass.

Be careful, however, that your tube is not too large. If rotation of the tube does not work, remove the tube and try a smaller size. Never force it through. The cricoid ring is the smallest diameter of the child's airway. In adults the smallest diameter lies between the vocal cords. This means that a tube too large for the child might pass through the vocal cords but not the cricoid ring. Never force an endotracheal tube down a pediatric airway. If the tube will not pass easily, choose a smaller size.

Be gentle in all of your manipulations. Pediatric airways are small and delicate and as such are prone to edema. A comparison to the adult illustrates the relative danger. The typical adult airway is 8 mm in diameter or greater. One mm of circumferential edema from intubation trauma leaves an airway of 6 mm diameter, a 25% reduction. An infant's airway typically is 3 mm in diameter. One mm circumferential edema here leaves an airway 1 mm in diameter, a 68% reduction. Even minimal trauma can create life threatening airway obstruction.

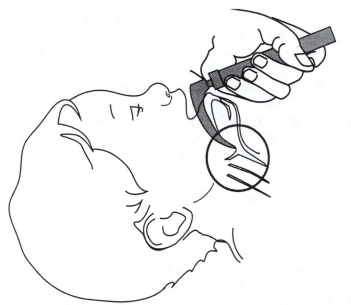

Fig. 9-4. A curved blade will sometimes fold the epiglottis down, hiding your view of the vocal cords.

Equipment for Pediatric Intubation

You will need the same type of equipment for the pediatric as for the adult intubation. The main difference to recognize is that the younger children are, the more different their anatomy is from the adult.

Pediatric carts need Miller blades in sizes 0 (premature), 1 (infant), and 2 (child). You can intubate a small child using a large blade, even an adult blade, by inserting the blade to the minimum depth needed to see the larynx. When using such a large blade you must shift the tongue to the left as far as possible. Otherwise the blade will fill the small mouth and leave you with no room to maneuver. Intubating a larger child with a blade that is too short may be impossible. Always try to have the correct size blade available for use.

Unexpected difficulties in intubation may arise. While not needed for the intubation itself, you should always have the correct size available for the child. Have a large suction catheter for clearing the mouth of secretions and vomit. and also need one which will go down the smallest endotracheal tube you might use.

Predict the correct size endotracheal tube before you start the intubation. Have both the next larger and next smaller sizes available in case you need them (Table 9-2).

We don't routinely use cuffed endotracheal tubes in children less than about 9 years old. Children's airways are small and cuffs take up space. Avoiding cuffs allows the use of a larger diameter tube, thereby minimizing airway resistance and maximizing airway toilet. It also avoids the excess pressure on the mucosa that a cuff can cause.

Do you need to worry about aspiration? In the young child, the smallest diameter is the cricoid ring, a round hole. Therefore the proper size round tube should seal the larynx and prevent aspiration. In the adult, the smallest diameter is the triangular opening between the cords. Our adult tube needs a cuff to help seal off the surrounding space. A properly sized pediatric tube will allow an air leak at 15-20 cm of water pressure but will sustain a seal below this. The absence of a leak means too large a tube, which may cause mucosal trauma and edema. The presence of a leak below 15-20 cm water pressure means too small a tube, increasing the risk of aspiration and possibly inadequate ventilation.

Intubating the Infant

The infant's head lies naturally in the sniffing position due to the prominence of the occiput. In fact, sometimes the occiput seems too high. The larynx falls too low to see easily. In such cases place a small hand towel or similar thickness object underneath the infant's shoulders. This raises the rest of the body and straightens the airway. The occiput tends to roll in the infant, making the act of balancing the head on your blade a challenge. Don't hesitate to have an assistant hold the head for you if you have problems. A small "donut" under the head or rolled towel placed on either side of the head serves the same purpose. With practice, balancing the head becomes second nature.

Open the mouth with your right index finger and thumb as far to the right side of the mouth as possible. Extend the head slightly as you do so. Avoid hyperextension which can obstruct the infant airway. The infant's mouth is so small compared to your hand that failure to place your fingers on the right will block your view. It can prevent insertion of the blade.

Carefully insert your blade into the child's mouth with your left hand and advance the blade until you see the epiglottis. Pick up the epiglottis gently with your blade and lift the mandible upward (Fig. 9-5). Sweep the tongue to the left

Table 9-2. Suggested sizes for pediatric endotracheal tubes:

Age	Size
Premature	2.5-3.5 mm I.D.
Newborn	3.5 mm I.D.
3-12 months	4.0 mm I.D.
1-2 years	4.5 mm I.D.
over 2 years	$4.5 + (\text{age in years} \div 4)$
French size, over 2 years	age in years + 18
Insertion depth to mid trachea	$12 + (\text{age in years} \div 2)$

as you do so. Avoid pressing on the upper gum line as you lift. The infant tongue is much larger relative to the mouth and mandible than the adult. Failure to sweep the tongue to the left will leave no room for visualization or for passage of the tube. A common error in children is to insert the blade too deep, into the esophagus. If you cannot see anatomy that you recognize then gently and under direct vision pull the blade tip back. Often the larynx will fall into view.

Figure 9-5 also demonstrates a way for you to provide your own cricoid pressure and manipulation of the trachea of a small infant. Use your fifth or little finger to gently push the larynx into position as you lift.

Pick up the chosen tube with the right hand and pass it through the vocal cords as you are watching. Stop when you see the double ring marking pass the cords. Carefully remove your laryngoscope blade. Be sure that the tube lies in the trachea by listening to the chest as described earlier. The small size of the infant allows easy transmission of sound. As my teachers used to say, you can hear breath sounds over a child's foot. Therefore, be especially careful to listen over the stomach and the chest to be certain that the tube is down the right hole. Another important factor is that the trachea of the infant is very short. Mainstem intubation is easy and fairly common. Make sure that you hear breath sounds on both sides of the chest before and after you secure the tube. Can you see the chest move on both sides? Note the depth marking on the tube in relationship to the gum line and compare it to the calculated depth. The infant trachea is so short compared to the adult that changing the head position can lead to a mainstem intubation or an extubation. Raising the chin raises the tube away from the carina, lowering the chin lowers the tube toward the carina. "The hose follows the nose" is a useful mnemonic.

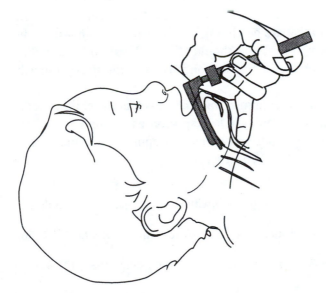

Fig. 9-5. Place head in neutral position. If needed, apply cricoid pressure using the little finger.

Infants can't hold their breaths as long as an adult can before the onset of hypoxia. Their functional residual capacity, that part of the lung storing oxygen, is small relative to their body size. Their metabolic rate is almost double that of an adult. If you experience difficulty with the intubation of an infant, stop the intubation and ventilate the child before proceeding with another attempt. *Lack of ventilation hurts patients, not the lack of an endotracheal tube.*

Intubating the Child

Gather the appropriate sizes of laryngoscope blades, endotracheal tubes, and ancillary equipment before approaching the child. Having it available before you start allows for greater flexibility and faster intubation.

Most children younger than 9 years old do not need a head roll to lift them into the sniffing position. However, look at the child and individualize the need based on the child's anatomy. You now know the angles that you need to bring the airway into a straight line.

The older the child, the more like an adult he or she will be. The child has some additional problems, however, that the infant lacks.

Children frequently have enlarged tonsils and adenoids. The tonsils sometimes meet or "kiss" in the midline and make visualization of the larynx a challenge. When faced with "kissing" tonsils, take your time while placing the laryngoscope blade. Avoid traumatizing the posterior pharynx. Tonsils are very friable tissue and can bleed easily.

If you can't intubate with the first attempt, withdraw, ventilate the child, and try again. Forewarned is forearmed. Check for missing teeth after you finish. You should look for any teeth that are newly missing. Often the tooth will lie in the posterior pharynx. If it isn't there, you should take an X-ray to be sure that the tooth isn't in the trachea or obstructing a bronchus. A tooth in the stomach will eventually pass.

The basic thing to remember when intubating a child is that the child is not a miniature adult. The anatomy and the physiologic responses to stress are different. Always take these factors into account when you approach a child. You'll make intubation easier and safer for all concerned.

Further Reading

Browning DH, Graves SA: Incidence of aspiration with endotracheal tubes in children. *J. Pediatr.* 1983; 102: 582

Koka BV, Jeon JM, et.al.: Postextubation croup in children. *Anesth. Analg.* 1977; 56: 501

Gregory GA: *Pediatric Anesthesia.* New York. Churchill-Livingstone, 1983, 437-439.

10 NASAL INTUBATION TECHNIQUES

N asal intubation is a useful technique to learn because it's sometimes the only safe way to intubate the patient.

Indications and Contraindications

You may prefer a nasal intubation for:

1. ease of patient positioning — placed awake so the patient can turn himself prone, etc.;

2. long-term intubation, as in the ICU — nasal tubes are better tolerated, less tube movement;

3. surgical access — nasal placement avoids surgical site in oral surgery, some facial fractures;

4. minimize risk of aspiration — awake placement when there is risk of emesis, GI bleeding, bowel obstruction;

5. difficult airway — awake intubation for short neck, morbid obesity, congenital anomaly, fractured mandible, inability to open mouth or move neck;

6. unstable cervical spine — awake intubation to identify symptoms during intubation, document neurologic status after intubation, avoid extension of neck during intubation;

7. unstable hemodynamic status — awake for ICU or CCU patients in shock to avoid the risk of hypotension due to general anesthesia or sedation;

We use nasal intubation frequently for emergency intubations in patients who are hemodynamically unstable, at risk for aspiration, or with anticipated difficult airways. You can perform awake oral intubations in all of the above situations. However, nasal intubations are often easier to perform and more comfortable for the awake patient than oral intubations.

Nasal intubations are also very useful for patients who must be intubated in awkward positions, such as pinned behind the steering wheel of their car, or unable to lay supine due to severe dyspnea in that position.

Nasal intubations are contraindicated in patients with nasal fractures or basilar skull fractures. The risk of causing more damage or of intubating the brain through a fractured ethmoid sinus is too high. They are relatively contraindicated with a history of nose bleeds and sinusitis. Unavoidable inflammation and edema from the tube can cause a recurrence of bleeding and infection.

Anatomy

Successful nasal intubation depends on an understanding of the anatomy of the nasopharynx. The nasal passages are not just open cylinders. Inside each nasal passage there are 3 bones which project inward from the lateral walls like shelves. These are the superior, middle, and inferior turbinates. Each turbinate consists of thin, spongy bone curled upon itself like a scroll and covered with mucous membrane. They serve to protect the openings of the sinuses. They also increase the surface area inside the nose to allow warming, humidification, and cleansing of inhaled air (Fig. 10-1).

During nasal intubation, the turbinates can be torn or otherwise damaged. Serious nose bleed can result. Sometimes the nasotracheal tracheal tube must be maneurvered past these potential obstructions.

It's important to remember that the nasal passages are perpendicular to the plain of the face. In other words, they are parallel to the floor when the patient is upright and the head is in a neutral position.

Behind the nasal passages lies the mucous membrane of the nasopharynx. This capillary rich bed allows the mucosa to shrink or expand in response to changes in heat, humidity, or allergens to protect the respiratory tract. It will also swell in response to trauma, infection including colds, and from crying. Swollen mucosa is more likely to bleed.

Techniques

Blind Nasal Intubation, Spontaneous Ventilation

Successful awake nasal intubations also start with assessment of the anatomy. To detect obstruction, pinch off each nostril in turn and then feel the

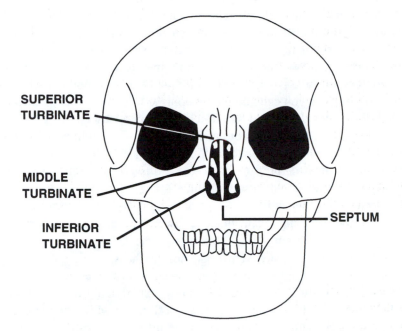

Fig. 10-1. Nasal anatomy. The inside of the nose is not smooth. Take care to avoid damaging the turbinates.

amount of air exhaled through the other. Look for septal deviation. Avoid the effected side of the nose if there is a history of nose bleeds and sinusitis.

You can perform nasal intubations with the patient either awake or asleep. For awake placement the patient must breath spontaneously.

Awake intubation is more difficult in a poorly prepared patient. This preparation can be as simple as topicalizing the nose and talking to the patient or as complex as injected nerve blocks and intravenous sedation. The approach will differ depending on where the intubation is performed.

For example, sedation should be used with extreme caution, if at all, in the field, where the patient's status may be deteriorating and the resources to manage potential complications are minimal. The hypoxic or exhausted patient may lose consciousness or become apneic with little warning. Numbing the trachea in a patient at risk for vomiting and aspiration is relatively contraindicated. The safe use of sedatives and local anesthetic topicalization depends on the clinical situation and the constant reassessment of the patient.

Some simple preparation of the nose, however, will improve patient comfort and cooperation, and hence patient safety. Several methods exist. We'll concentrate here on methods which can be also be used in the field. More complex regimens needing special equipment, skills, and time will be discussed in detail in Chapter 15 and 16.

Use a nasal vasoconstrictor, such as phenylephrine, to reduce the risk of nose bleeds during nasal intubation — even if you don't have time to wait for peak effect. All local anesthetics, except cocaine, cause vasodilation. Vasodilation produces edema, narrows the opening, and makes nosebleeds more likely. Vasoconstrictors aid tube passage and minimize bleeding. You can either use a nasal spray or drops or you can add phenylephrine to your topical solution.

The use of 5% cocaine liquid solution also vasoconstricts, but is often unavailable. Lidocaine gel is fairly liquid and easily "sniffed," while the ointment is viscous and must be allowed time to melt.

Unless contraindicated, prepare both sides. this allows you to switch sides immediately if the first side is unsuccessful.

Use a plastic IV catheter (Fig. 10-2), such as an 18-20g, to spray 2 cc of 4% lidocaine onto the nasopharyngeal mucosa toward the posterior superior aspect of each nasal passage (total 4 cc). This numbs the back of the nasal passage which can be difficult to reach. This also numbs the sphenopalatine ganglion, the network of nerves supplying in part the nose and nasopharynx.

Alternatively, combine one cc of one percent phenylephrine with four cc of viscous lidocaine. Dribble the mixture down both nares while the patient sniffs. You can also use cetacaine spray to numb the nose but warn the patient that it will sting for about 10 to 20 seconds. Always keep track of the total dose of local anesthetic given since absorption through the mucous membrane is rapid and toxicity can occur.

I frequently pass progressively larger nasal airways coated with local

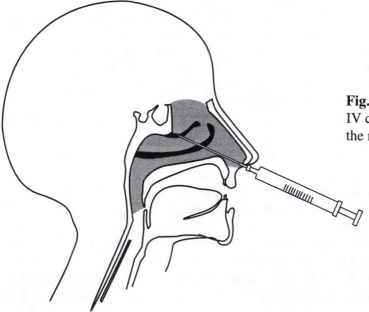

Fig. 10-2. Use of an IV catheter to numb the nose.

anesthetic ointment. I personally don't believe that this practice further dilates the nasal passage. However, this practice does enhance the numbing. It also tests the passage for size and evidence of obstruction. Meanwhile, the patient becomes accustomed to the passage of nasal tubes, making passage of the larger endotracheal tube more tolerable.

Nasal topicalization can be accompanied by a nerve block of the glossopharyngeal or superior laryngeal nerves as desired.

Simply telling the patient what to expect improves cooperation. Constantly monitor level of consciousness and adequacy of ventilation and oxygenation.

One of the advantages of nasal intubation is that it is more easily performed than oral intubations when the patient is in an awkward positions. The best position for the head is still the sniffing position. Use a bit more flexion than extension. Extreme extension makes the angle that the tube must turn to enter the trachea more acute. Placing the patient in a semi-sitting position, if not contraindicated, prevents the tongue and soft tissue from falling over the larynx and can make intubation easier. This can also make it easier for the patient to breathe.

Warming the tube in hot water makes it more pliable and easier to pass. Coat the tip of the tube with local anesthetic ointment. If none is at hand then any water soluble lubricant or even plain water can serve. Make sure the lubricant does not enter the tube itself.

Stabilize the patient head with your non-dominant hand and use your other hand to slide the tube straight back into the nose, perpendicular to the face, and parallel to the floor of the nose (Fig. 10-3a) . Avoid the common tendency to thread the tube into the frontal sinus, a painful maneuver likely to cause a nosebleed. Be gentle, because the middle turbinate is fragile in most patients and can be fractured or torn.

Keep the bevel turned toward the septum. This will make it less likely to tear the mucosa or damage a turbinate. For the right nares, the tube concavity will be turned toward the feet. When using the left nares, this means that the concavity will be turned toward the top of the head. The left sided tube will need to be rotated 180° once it has entered the posterior pharynx so that it's natural curvature aims it toward the laryngeal opening.

Advance the tube until you feel a give or loss of resistance; the tube has just turned the corner into the posterior pharynx (Fig. 10-3b). Unless your patient is too exhausted or weak, they will be startled. Calmly explain to them what is happening. This loss of resistence is often quite abrupt and may be accompanied by a crunching sensation as the tube passes the turbinates. Gentleness and avoidance of force will help to avoid trauma and nose bleeds. If you meet resistance, slowly twist the tube while applying *gentle* forward pressure. The tube will often slide past the obstruction. Never force the tube or the tube tip may dissect under the mucous membrane into the retropharyngeal space or rip a turbinate.

If you can't pass the tube easily and gentle twisting of the tube fails to solve the problem, then either switch to the other nares or try a smaller tube.

Now slowly advance the tube during the patient's inspiration, when the vocal cords are most open. Listen to the breath sounds through the tube. As long as the tube and the trachea are aligned you will hear hollow, loud breath sounds and see condensation inside the tube. Continue to advance the tube. If the tube continues to advance and you still hear breath sounds the tube is in the trachea (Fig. 10-3c). Successful placement often makes the patient cough. If cervical spine precautions are being used, your assistant needs to be prepared to steady the head and upper torso to prevent movement during this time.

Check immediately that you have actually intubated the patient. Inflate the cuff and check for the presence of bilateral breath sounds. With the patient breathing spontaneously, you will feel the air moving in and out of the tube. When she ventilates spontaneously you'll feel the bag collapse with each breath. She won't be able to speak once the tube passes between the cords and the cuff

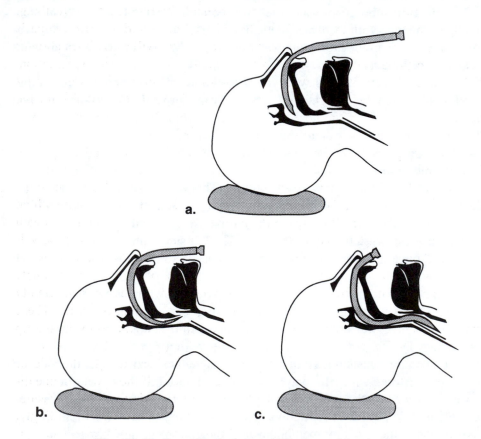

a.

b.   c.

Fig. 10-3a, b, c. Technique of blind nasal intubation.

is inflated. Condensation will form inside the tube as she breathes. When you ventilate the patient the chest rises as you squeeze the bag.

Make sure that the breath sounds are bilateral and equal. If there is a main-stem intubation slowly pull the tube back until bilateral breath sounds reappear. Depth markings on the tube for a nasal intubation will be about 27–28 cm at the nares in the average adult.

I believe that the cuff should always be inflated once the patient is intubated. Sometimes people leave the cuff deflated so that the patient can talk around the tube. I believe that this risks aspiration. The tube holds the cords apart and de-feats the normal protective mechanisms. Secretions can dribble down the out-side of the tube into the trachea.

Once you verify endotracheal placement, suction down the tube to clear any secretions, blood, or tissue that may be present. Aspiration can occur during na-sal intubation, even in awake patients. A suction catheter should pass easily through the gentle curve of the nasotracheal tube. If it doesn't, the tube may be crimped in its path through the posterior pharynx.

Crimping partially obstructs the tube, increasing the resistance to breathing. It also impairs the ability to keep the tube cleared of secretions. If the tube is crimped, pulling it out or pushing it in a small amount will sometimes allow it to curve more smoothly. Be careful to avoid extubation or mainstem intubation. If the tube still won't allow passage of a suction catheter consider replacing it with either a larger tube or an oral tube at the earliest safe opportunity for the patient.

Managing Difficult Passage of the Tube

Sometimes the tube won't pass easily. As long as the tip of the tube is aligned with the trachea then breath sounds are present as you advance the tube. If the tube passes into the esophagus, breath sounds vanish. The patient with no topical anesthesia frequently gags. Stop, pull the tube back until you hear breath sounds again, then slowly advance once more. If the tube tip catches in the val-lecula or one of the piriform sinuses, you'll hear good breath sounds, but won't be able to advance the tube. Changing either the angle of the head or the angle of the tube will often bring the tube into alignment with the trachea. Gently twist the tube a bit as you advance. Try flexing or extending the head. These maneuvers change the angle of the endotracheal tube and frequently let the tip slide off the obstruction and into the trachea.

If the tube won't enter the trachea easily, turn the head toward the side or change the degree of flexion or extension (Fig. 10-4a-c). If movement in one di-rection doesn't work, turn it the other way. Try applying cricoid pressure. Picture where you're aiming the tip of the tube and adjust the head accordingly. A tube placed in the right nostril tends to cross to the left lower pharynx. Therefore, moving the head slightly to the right of midline for a right-sided tube will align the trachea with the tube. For left nasal intubations move the head to the left. Pushing the larynx toward the side opposite the nares being used can also help. Any manipulation of the head must take into account the patient's risk of existing cervical spinal injury.

Having the awake patient stick out the tongue can occasionally clear a path to the larynx.

Sometimes further topicalization or sedation will smooth the intubation. However, you must weigh the risks of these maneuvers against the benefits. A sedated patient with a numb larynx can aspirate easily.

As mentioned earlier, submucosal dissection can occur if the tip of the tube tears the mucosa and slides underneath it. Suspect that this has occured if you

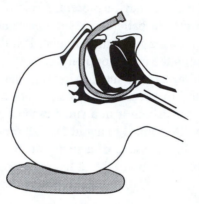

a. ENDOTRACHEAL TUBE CAUGHT IN THE VALLECULA

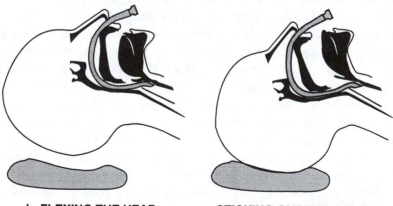

b. FLEXING THE HEAD　　　**c. STICKING OUT THE TONGUE**

Fig. 10-4. If the tube tip stops in the valecula, or the piriform sinus, flex the head slightly or have the patient open her mouth and stick her tongue out. Both change the angle of the tube.

can't hear breath sounds once the tube has entered the posterior pharynx or if you feel a lot of resistance as you advance the tube. The conscious patient often complains of severe pain when this happens. With submucosal dissection you won't see the tube in the posterior pharynx but you will see a bulge behind the tonsillar pillars. When a nasotracheal tube is submucosal, remove it carefully. Be prepared for a heavy nosebleed. If nasal intubation is still indicated, try the other side and proceed carefully. You may need to consider postponing elective surgery because of the risk of retropharyngeal hematoma and abscess formation. A patient who already has airway obstruction could have worsening of the obstruction due to the increased swelling.

Adjunctive Techniques to Nasal Intubation

The use of a type of nasotracheal tube called an Endotrol tube can facilitate nasal intubations. Nasotracheal tubes sometimes enter the esophagus because they won't curve forward enough after entering the oropharynx. Endotrol tubes solve this problem with a pull cord attached to a ring near the 15mm adaptor. Pulling the ring turns the tip of the tube anteriorly, allowing you to manipulate the tip with more precise control.

A device called a BAAM, or Beck Airway Airflow Monitor, can make the breath sounds which are so critical to success, easier to hear even in noisy environments. The BAAM is a small, cylindrical, plastic whistle which fits over the 15 mm adapter for the endotracheal tube. The device is about the small size as an endotracheal tube adaptor and is disposible. A whistle is produced whenever the patient inhales or exhales through the tube when the BAAM is attached. Even very low amounts of airflow will produce a whistle. The whistle is said to be loud enough to hear in an ambulance or helicopter.

The pitch varies both with the breathing cycle and with the position of the tube tip relative to the larynx because the airflow velocity through the device changes. The provider can use the loudness of the whistle and the pitch to more precisely guide the tube.

The BAAM has also been used to assist difficult oral intubations. Spontaneous respirations or an assistant's gentle pushing on the chest produce a guiding whistle.

Since minimal movement of air produces a whistle, the BAAM has been used in some very unique situations, including CPR, where chest compressions caused sufficient airflow to produce a whistle. While not optimal, it may be a useful adjunct for those situations when the conventional approach isn't possible.

The BAAM should not be left in position for more than 2 minutes at a time following successful intubation since its small aperture of 2mm would produce excessive resistence to breathing.

When the conventional tube won't pass blindly, you can use your laryngoscope to visualize the larynx (Fig. 10-5). I usually use a curved blade for this maneuver. It gives me more room to manipulate the tube. Once you see the larynx hold your left hand firmly in position. You can often push the tube forward yourself and direct it into the larynx. If the tube is still by passing the cords you can have an assistant push the tube into the trachea while you guide the tip of the tube with magill forceps or some other instrument. Your assistant must position himself to avoid blocking your view. Grab either the tip of the tube or the area behind the cuff. Never grab the cuff itself with your forceps. You can easily rip it, leaving no way to seal off the trachea. Use this combined technique on either awake or anesthetized patients. The technique can also be used in the apneic patient. You can use a bent stylet or a hook to curve the endotracheal tube anteriorly if you don't have Magill forceps.

Sometimes the endotracheal tube aims at the larynx but won't enter. A firm catheter passed through the endotracheal tube when it's lined up may enter the trachea and provide a guide to insert the tube. Nasogastric tubes or tube exchangers are useful for this purpose. Soft suction catheters can also serve if long enough. Firmly hold the endotracheal tube at the point where breath sounds are most audible, then pass the catheter through the tube. Slide the tube over the catheter into the larynx. Remove the catheter and check breath sounds (Fig. 10-6).

Fiberoptic bronchoscopy is often combined with nasotracheal intubation. The bronchoscope can act as the ultimate guide since it allows you to enter the larynx under direct vision to direct your tube into the trachea. This technique is discussed in detail in Chapter 13.

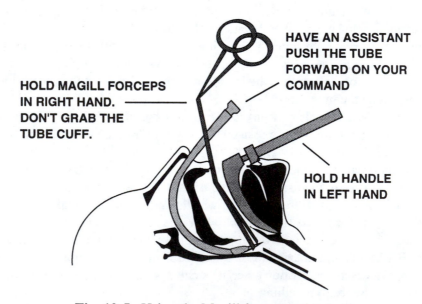

HAVE AN ASSISTANT PUSH THE TUBE FORWARD ON YOUR COMMAND

HOLD MAGILL FORCEPS IN RIGHT HAND. DON'T GRAB THE TUBE CUFF.

HOLD HANDLE IN LEFT HAND

Fig. 10-5. Using the Magill forceps to intubate.

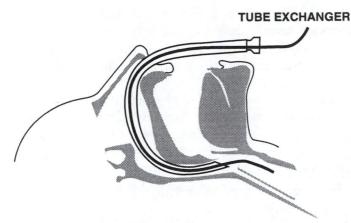

Fig. 10-6. Using a tube exchanger to assist intubation.

One final caveat with the combined oral/nasal technique. Sometimes you can't see the trachea during direct laryngoscopy. If the patient is breathing, listen for breath sounds as you pass the tube. By using their loudness to guide your aim you can blindly intubate a patient during direct laryngoscopy.

Patient Safety

Constantly monitor the patient to ensure adequate respiration, airway protection, and hemodynamic stability during naotracheal intubation. Use suction frequently. Check oxygen saturation if you have it.

Provide supplemental oxygen if available. This can be administered through nasal prongs, a face mask, or simple oxygen tubing placed near the patient's mouth.

A nasal airway can also be placed in the opposite nostril and hooked up to oxygen. The patient's respirations can even be supported with an Ambu bag as long as the mouth is closed (see Fig. 3-4.). This is a very useful technique during the administration of anesthesia because the depth of the anesthetic can be maintained in an anesthetized patient. Be aware that the tip of the canula can deflect the nasotracheal tube away from the larynx if it's long enough. If you think this is happening then withdraw the airway slightly and try again.

Emergency Treatment of Nosebleed

When a nose bleed occurs during nasal intubation the treatment depends on its severity as well as on the clinical situation.

If the bleeding is minimal, it may be best to leave the endotracheal tube in place and continue with the attempt. The tube will actually allow you to provide more pressure to the site. On the other hand, if bleeding is severe enough to cause blood to accumulate in the posterior pharynx, then the tube should probably be removed and pressure applied to pinch the nostril on that side firmly closed against the septum. Suction the oropharynx frequently. You may have to position the patient in trendelenburg or on the side to allow blood to pool away from the larynx.

Ventilation and intubation attempts will be more difficult, however, securing the airway in the apneic or respiratory distressed patient will be crucial to preventing aspiration or hypoventilation. Other emergency measures to control a severe nose bleed — while awaiting assistance from a head and neck or emergency specialist — include inflating the cuff from an endotracheal tube or the balloon from a foley catheter inside the nose and nasopharynx to compress the site.

A Laryngeal Mask Airway (LMA) may be useful in the emergency situation of severe nosebleed in a patient with an unprotected airway who can't be intubated. Since the bleeding comes from above, the LMA can help seal off the glottis and allow ventilation. An LMA, however, won't prevent aspiration. Constantly monitor the patient. (See Chapter 13 for more on LMAs.)

Further Reading

Click M: Airway another way: blind nasotracheal intubation. *JEMS*. Feb 1996: 58-63

Pederson B: Blind nasotracheal intubation: A review and a new guided technique. *Acta. Anaesth. Scandinav.* 1971; 15: 107

Stene JK, Cook RT, Beck GP: Blind nasal, blind oral and digital intubation in trauma patients: use of the Beck Airway Airflow Monitor. =*Anesthesiology News.* March 1996; 35-39

11 STUDIES IN DIFFICULT INTUBATIONS: TRICKS OF THE TRADE

Most intubations proceed without difficulty. Certain patients, however, are difficult to intubate by virtue of their anatomy or the circumstances of the intubation. Unfortunately, such patients can also be difficult to ventilate, creating a double quandary. With experience you learn to anticipate these difficult intubations. This allows you to avoid problems by altering technique at the start. Let's look at some of the more common difficult intubations and some of the tricks of the trade.

One word of caution. Difficulty in intubation, especially when accompanied by difficulty in ventilation, is a life threatening situation. Even experienced intubators seek help when they have trouble. Inexperienced intubators are well advised to have an experienced intubator standing by during the intubation. This can save precious time in an emergency. The more experienced person can also give you pointers on correcting your technique.

Cardiac Arrest

Cardiac arrest victims are often challenging intubations because of the circumstances surrounding the intubation. Excitement and apprehension accompany this life saving effort. If you don't intubate very often, you'll be very nervous. Even experienced intubators get excited in emergency situations. We control our excitement and let the adrenalin work for us rather than against us. **Step one**, therefore, is to remain in control of your own excitement.

Step two is to quickly assess the situation. Is the patient being ventilated? Is there suction available? What help do you have? What position is the patient in and how can you optimize that position?

You usually find the patient in one of two awkward positions. When the patient lies on the floor, you must intubate on your knees. Mechanical advantage is more difficult from this position. You must rely more heavily on your arm strength to lift the head rather than your upper back and shoulder muscles. The natural tendency to lean forward and bend your arm will make it hard for you to balance (Fig. 11-1). The weight of the patient pulls you forward when you try to lift. Instead, keep your left arm and your back as straight as you can. Tense your buttocks and thigh muscles to form a firm base of support, and lift upward (Fig. 11-2). Straddling the head with your knees allows you to steady

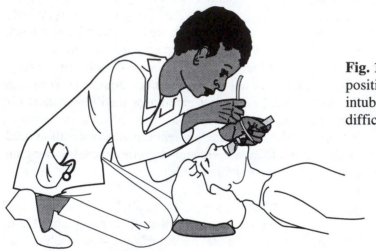

Fig. 11-1. Awkward positioning of intubator makes for difficult intubations.

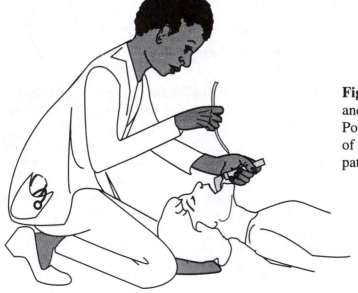

Fig. 11-2. Keep back and arm straight. Position your center of gravity over the patient's head.

the head, steady yourself, and improve your angle or approach. Remember that several folded sheets or towels under the head lift it into the sniffing position. Ask for help in lifting the head into position if you need it. Your head and shoulders should be over the patient's head. This improves your center of gravity during the lift.

Some anesthesiologists recommend lying prone on your stomach to intubate a patient on the floor. They place their weight on their elbows, eliminating the problem of balance and improving the angle of view.

Unfortunately, the second awkward position finds the patient in the typical hospital bed (Fig. 11-3, 11-4). Why is this awkward? First, most hospital beds have a fairly high headboard which prevents easy access to the patient's head. Have someone remove this headboard while you prepare your equipment.

Second, if you can't easily reach the patient, pull him or her toward the head of the bed. This only takes a moment, but for small individuals like myself it is a moment well spent. If you do not have to lean forward you will have more effective mechanical advantage and control.

Third, you'll often find the patient on a soft hospital mattress with the hard cardiac arrest board under his back. Because this allows effective CPR, we take

Fig. 11-3. Problems with intubation in the bed: awkward angle, headboard in the way, backboard makes head angle severe, CPR moves the patient.

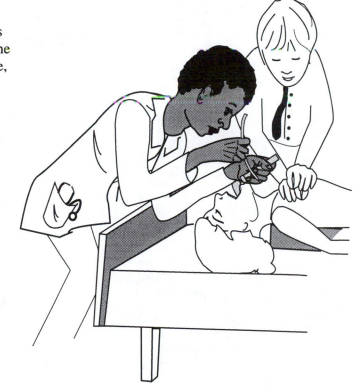

this position for granted. We often fail to notice that the patient's head now hangs fully extended off the back of the board. A look at the angles that this produces shows that you must lift the patient's head much higher to straighten the airway (Fig. 11-5). Lifting a heavy head high under these conditions is quite

Fig. 11-4. Optimize your position during CPR: remove headboard, move patient closer to head of bed, place head in sniffing position, stop CPR during attempt, keep back and arm straight.

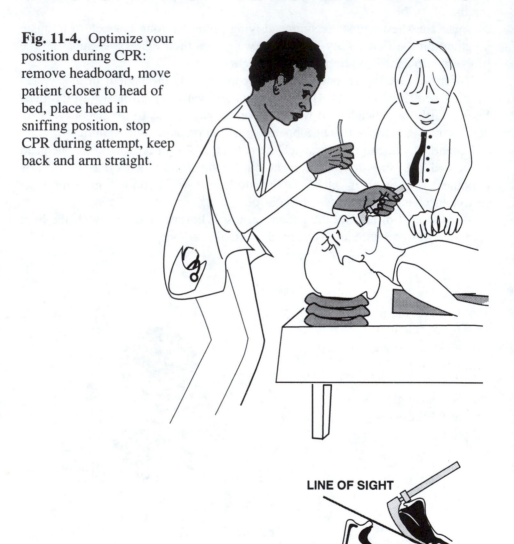

LINE OF SIGHT

Fig. 11-5. Overextension of the head makes the larynx appear more anterior on laryngoscopy.

difficult. Use pillows to put the head in the sniffing position and decrease the lift you need. Don't hesitate to ask for assistance in lifting or in maintaining lift while you place the tube. Cricoid pressure to push the larynx down into view can also help in situations like this (Fig. 11-6, 11-7).

Fourth, CPR means that someone is forcefully pushing on the patient's chest. The patient and bed are both moving up and down. Moving targets are hard to hit at the best of times. I usually get in position, visualize the larynx, and try to pass the tube. If the movement prevents this, I ask for momentary discontinuation of CPR. Yell "stop CPR." Pass the tube. Yell "begin CPR." This should take no longer than 15 to 20 seconds, usually less. If you have any difficulty passing the tube have your associates begin CPR again. Remove your blade, and ventilate the patient. Try again. Never delay CPR for an extended period because of an intubation attempt.

Always remember that adequate ventilation is more important than intubation. If you have difficulty, stop and ventilate the patient while you decide what you must try next.

Following intubation, suction the tube and trachea carefully to remove any secretions and blood aspirated during the resuscitation.

Obesity

Patients with obesity or with short, muscular necks can sometimes be hard to intubate (Fig. 11-8). Excess soft tissue around the larynx and decreased hyoid/mentum distance hinder displacement of those tissues forward by the

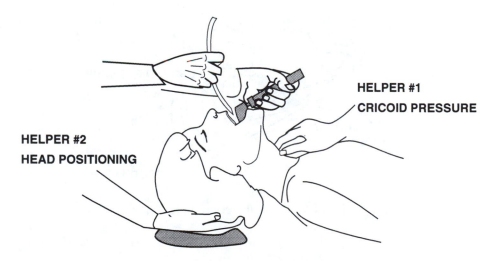

Fig. 11-6. The use of helpers.

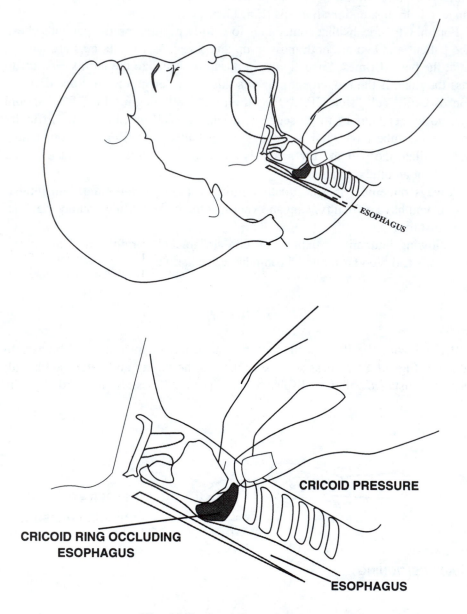

ESOPHAGUS

CRICOID PRESSURE

CRICOID RING OCCLUDING ESOPHAGUS

ESOPHAGUS

Fig. 11-7. Applying cricoid pressure.

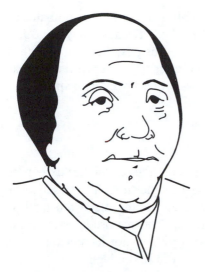

Fig. 11-8. The obese patient often has a short, thick neck and much tissue under the skin.

laryngoscope blade. Without such displacement the larynx may not be visible. Excess soft tissue collapsing over the laryngeal structures may make manual ventilation   difficult. Techniques for difficult ventilation are discussed in Chapters 3 and 13.

I usually make the first attempt at intubation with the blade I am most comfortable with. In emergency situations I often choose a Macintosh curved blade. In my opinion, its broader flange is more forgiving of less than perfect placement and awkward positioning — conditions common in the emergency. It also makes balancing the patient's head easier in those circumstances. However, in obese patients or those with an "anterior" airway, the curved blade sometimes won't give you good visualization. It doesn't allow enough displacement of tissue forward in these cases and the larynx remains hidden. Therefore, if I can't see the larynx with the Mac on the first try in this patient group, then I switch to a straight blade. The straight blade doesn't rely as heavily on the ability to displace the tissues of the hypopharynx forward. It flattens them.

The straight blade has another advantage. Inserting the curved blade can be difficult in the obese patient because the chest can get in the way of the handle. The straight blade bypasses this problem. Substituting a short laryngoscope handle often works as well.

Through the Veil:
Partial Plates and Cleft Palates

Patients will sometimes have missing upper front teeth. These patients pose a peculiar problem for intubation. Beginners frequently get a superb view of the larynx, they just can't pass the tube. The absence of teeth allows the intubator to see the larynx without lifting the mandible (Fig. 11-9). Because they have not opened the patient's mouth enough they can't get the tube past the teeth on either side. The solution is to lift the jaw upward even after you can see the larynx. Don't try to pass the tube through the gap. There usually is not enough space.

Edentulous

The same situation described above can occur here. You see the larynx before the mouth is open wide enough to allow passage of the tube. The absence of teeth on the mandible sometimes changes the angle of the blade during lift. Usually, however, the change in "feel" and balance that this produces is minimal. It is often offset by the relief of the intubator about not having to worry about the teeth. Intubation is easier without teeth if you lift enough.

Receding Chin

Patients with receding chins, caused by hypoplastic mandibles, often have very "anterior airways" (Fig. 11-10). There is frequently not enough room to displace the tissue forward when you intubate. You may need to do an awake intubation if the chin is extremely hypoplastic. You should anticipate the need for cricoid pressure and a straight blade.

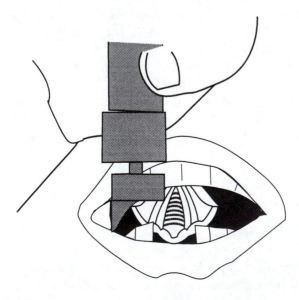

Fig. 11-9. You can see the larynx because the teeth are missing, even though the mouth is not wide enough to pass the tube.

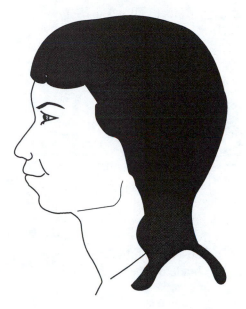

Fig. 11-10. Patients with hypoplastic mandibles, or receding chins, often have very anterior larynxes.

Overbites

The upper teeth in a prominent overbite will get in the way of a Macintosh blade (Fig. 11-11). You must follow the curve of the tongue into the mouth to insert a curved blade. The higher vertical profile of this blade may bump into the teeth if you don't open the mouth as much as possible. Straight blades avoid these problems.

Lift straight upward on these patients. You can easily push on the teeth if you use your laryngoscope as a lever. There are two tricks to try if you can't see. The first is cricoid pressure, a handy standby anytime you have difficulty seeing the larynx. The second is to substitute a shorter straight blade. You can sometimes insert a number one or two Miller blade inside the mouth such that the radius of any rotational movement of your blade occurs inside the radius of the teeth. This allows you to "lever" safely. If the blade is long enough, it can give you a better view.

Poor Neck Mobility

Poor neck mobility can occur for a number of reasons. Arthritic fusion of the vertebrae in older individuals often limits the range of motion. This limitation can be so severe that no extension or flexion of the head can occur. Torticollis or wry neck prevents full range of motion. Finally, trauma to the neck may limit

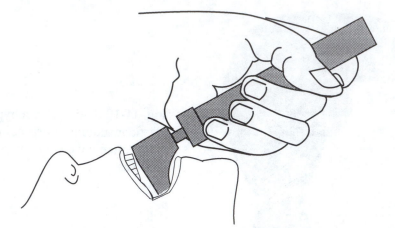

Fig. 11-11. In the presence of an overbite be careful to lift the jaw upward instead of rotating the blade on the teeth.

motion. In the latter case your patient may have a cervical collar or other restraint to prevent damage to the spinal cord.

It is often safest to intubate these patient awake. Techniques include the use of fiberoptic laryngoscopes and awake blind-nasal intubations. Sometimes the only safe choice is a tracheostomy. We'll discuss awake intubations later. For the moment let's assume that you have a patient with no neck mobility in need of intubation. He is unconscious or perhaps in cardiac arrest. What can you try?

First, let's discuss the patient with limited range of motion but *no* risk of spinal cord injury. When you can't extend the head you can't align the airway axes. The larynx looks very anterior during laryngoscopy (Fig. 11-12). Sometimes you can't even see the arytenoids. Lift the head as far off the bed as you can, suspending the head from your blade. This may be enough to bring the arytenoids into view. If it is, aim for the space immediately above the arytenoids, where the gap between the vocal cords lies. Straight blades often work better than curved blades in this situation. Forceful cricoid pressure may push the larynx down into view.

Make sure the stylet in your endotracheal tube has a **bend** on the end, shaping the tube like a hockey stick. Test to make sure that the stylet slides in and out easily despite the hook. Aim your tube anteriorly at the point where you think the larynx lies. Be gentle.

When you put a pronounced bend in the stylet, you sometimes find that the tube will not advance easily. The tip of the tube points upward, into the anterior wall of the trachea (Fig. 11-13). In this case you will feel resistance to pushing the tube in. Often the assistant holding cricoid pressure feels you pushing

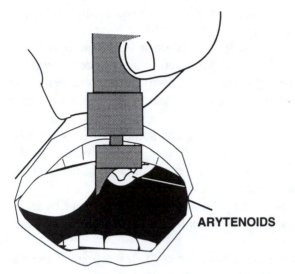

Fig. 11-12. The view seen with an anterior larynx. Here you can see the arytenoids. Often you see no landmarks.

ARYTENOIDS

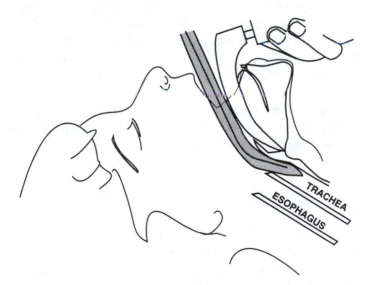

TRACHEA

ESOPHAGUS

Fig. 11-13. You may not be able to advance the tube if the stylet is bent to sharply. If this happens, slowly back the stylet out — then push the tube forward.

against the larynx. If this happens, fix your tube firmly in position and have someone else slowly remove the stylet from the tube. Advance the tube gently at the same time. Gently twisting the tube may allow the bevel to slip off the anterior commissure and slide down the trachea (Fig. 11-14).

If this fails and you feel you have the tube lined up with the laryngeal inlet there is another trick to try. Remove the stylet carefully. Advance a long and fairly firm suction catheter or nasogastric tube down the endotracheal tube while you hold it steady. Once inserted, use the catheter as a stylet to advance the endotracheal tube.

By aiming your tube at the likely location you can sometimes pass the tube into the larynx without seeing landmarks. If you do pass the tube blindly, make absolutely certain that you immediately test for proper tube placement. Tubes can easily slip into the esophagus in situations like this.

In the event that you can't intubate the patient, ventilate the patient by mask between attempts. Periodically suction the mouth and oropharynx for secretions. Ask for other intubators to try.

What do you do if you absolutely should not or can't flex or extend the patient's neck? When faced with the trauma patient in a halo, cervical collar, or other restraining device you face a difficult responsibility. You must secure the airway without injuring the patient. A halo device will keep the patient's head in a safe position. You may therefore try the techniques described above without further securing the head. Patients secured by sandbags or cervical collars must receive further protection. Have a knowledgeable assistant, the surgeon or neurosurgeon if present, hold the head and neck in a neutral position while you attempt intubation (Fig. 11-15). Lift the mandible upward, not the head and neck. Often you can see enough anatomy to allow intubation. If you can't intubate quickly, a tracheostomy may be the quickest and safest means of securing the airway. More extensive discussion of the management of the patient with potential cervical spine injury is found in Chapter 12.

Fixed Airway Obstruction

Airway obstruction is a life threatening emergency. Poor intubation technique may worsen airway obstruction, a potentially fatal situation. If you are an inexperienced intubator, you should summon and defer to the skill and judgement of any available experienced intubators. We often bring such patients to an operating room. There they are either intubated awake or under deep inhalational anesthesia with spontaneous ventilation. The personnel and means to perform emergency tracheostomy are immediately available and ready. Inexperienced intubators should not attempt intubation of an obstructed airway unless in their judgement only immediate intubation will save the patient's life.

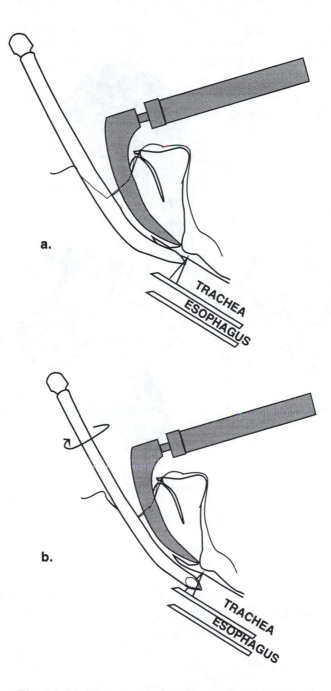

Fig. 11-14. The tube tip in **a** is caught on the anterior cummissure. Rotate the tube, as in **b**, to allow it to pass.

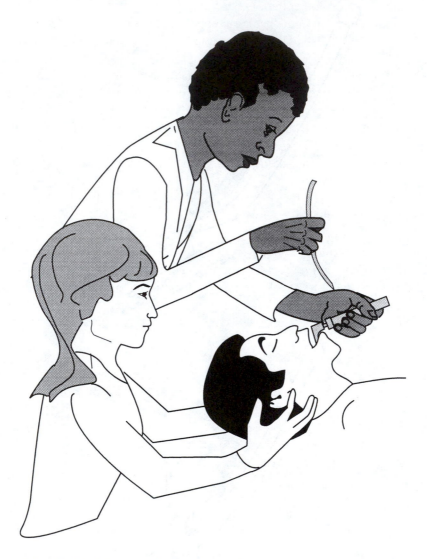

Fig. 11-15. When intubating the patient with possible neck injury have an assistant stabilize the head and neck. Lift only the mandible. Don't extend the head.

The most common emergencies involving airway obstruction include epiglottitis, croup, foreign body, trauma, and tumor. Epiglottis, croup, and foreign body are most common in the pediatric population but can occur in the adult.

When you initially evaluate these patients let them sit up if they're more comfortable breathing in this position and their vital signs are stable. A patient who is sitting has a larger functional residual capacity than one lying down — about 1 liter larger in the adult. In other words the lung volume used to exchange oxygen is larger. When a patient lies down, soft tissue around the airway tends to collapse over the airway, possibly increasing obstruction in the compromised patient. Also, sitting may slow the development of any edema.

Give them supplemental oxygen. Someone who can manage airway obstruction must accompany the patient if the patient needs to leave the emergency area. They should **never** be sent alone for special examinations, X-rays, or another facility. This intubator must take all the equipment needed for intubation and ventilation.

Don't subject a child to unnecessary laboratory exams or separate him prematurely from parents. Crying and screaming increases airway edema. Keep him calm. **Do not** sedate him. Sedation may cause him to lose what airway he has. Placing the parent in a wheelchair and the child in her lap may be the best choice for transporting a frightened child with airway obstruction around the hospital setting.

If the patient is dying and can't wait for more specialized help, you must proceed with caution. Call for the means to do cricothyrotomy or tracheostomy. Never paralyze or sedate a patient with airway obstruction unless in your judgement this is the only way to proceed safely. The muscle tone of the larynx may be the only factor maintaining the airway. The use of sedatives and muscle relaxants carries very high risk in this type of patient.

Gently visualize the larynx by direct laryngoscopy. Patients in extremis usually won't fight you as you do this. If you can identify landmarks, then intubate the patient. Use an endotracheal tube of appropriate size. By appropriate size I mean the largest one that will fit in the swollen airway. Don't try the largest one that should normally fit a patient of that size and age. Have a variety of tubes available, including the smallest pediatric tubes. I once used an infant sized number 3 endotracheal tube to intubate an 80 kg, 72 inch adult with epiglottitis because that was the only tube that would fit. Needless to say this woefully small tube was replaced by a surgical airway once the situation stabilized.

If you can't identify the anatomy, look for air bubbles coming from the larynx as a clue to the location of the cords. Have an assistant push on the chest if the patient isn't breathing. When the patient is breathing, give oxygen during the attempts by having an assistant blow oxygen into the mouth. Adequately ventilate with oxygen between attempts. Consider placement of a cricothyroid catheter to insufflate oxygen or the use a jet ventilator if hypoxia is present.

I advise the lone inexperienced intubator to stop after two or three attempts. Emergency cricothyrotomy or tracheostomy is indicated at this point.

Blood in the Oropharynx

Blood in the oropharynx predisposes the patient to aspiration and hypoxia. Fresh post operative cleft palates and tonsillectomies, severe nosebleeds, massive G.I. bleeders, and trauma victims are examples. In the worst case scenario, the patient is unconscious, unable to protect their airway, and is bleeding so badly that you can't see any landmarks at all. It's a frightening experience.

Handling the situation in an operating room where there is lighting, equipment, personnel, and experienced intubators makes sense. Life threatening emergencies sometimes force less than optimal circumstances.

Suction the airway frequently or continuously. This topic is discussed in detail in Chapter 12.

The Use of Cricoid Pressure

Cricoid pressure is one of the most valuable aides you have during a difficult intubation. We use it not only to improve visualization of the so-called anterior airway, but also to help prevent aspiration. To apply cricoid pressure, place your thumb on one side of the cricoid ring and your index or ring finger on the other. Push down firmly. This forces the cricoid ring against the vertebral column and effectively seals the esophagus. It also forces the vocal cords downward and perhaps into the field of view (see again, Fig. 11-7).

To help protect from aspiration, the pressure must be applied to the cricoid ring. If the cricoid pressure is being applied to improve your view, visualization may be better if your assistant presses on the thyroid cartilage rather than the cricoid.

You'll frequently use cricoid pressure. However, you should recognize that even this technique has problems.

While very effective against passive regurgitation, you should release cricoid pressure when the patient actively vomits. The obstructed esophagus might rupture because of high pressure.

Also, no matter how useful cricoid pressure usually is, it will occasionally prevent passage of the endotracheal tube. Cricoid pressure will sometimes pinch a child's soft airway closed. Sometimes in an adult the angle created by the downward displacement is too acute, preventing entry of the tube. This is especially true when inexperienced helpers push on other parts of the larynx in addition to the cricoid or if they push the cricoid off to the side. If you are having a great deal of difficulty intubating, consider releasing part or all of the cricoid pressure to see if it helps.

Cricoid pressure should be used cautiously, if at all, when there is an upper airway foreign body or if there is risk of cervical spine injury.

A Difficult Intubation Algorithm

The patients described above may prove impossible for even an experienced intubator to intubate. If you anticipate a difficult elective intubation it's often best to plan an awake intubation from the outset. If intubation fails after inducing general anesthesia, you can wake the patient up and intubate him awake (Fig. 11-16). The techniques for awake intubation will be discussed in Chapter 15.

Awake intubation may not be an option in the emergency situation or in the unresponsive patient (Fig. 11-17). If you can adequately mask ventilate the patient then you have many options and time to explore them. Call for assistance. Rarely will you be in a situation where you are the only person trained in intubation. Never hesitate to ask for help. That help can be getting equipment ready, aid in holding the head or neck in position, or asking someone else to intubate. When faced with a difficult intubation you should call for backup, if such backup exists. Backup can be an anesthesiologist, any other intubator, or a surgeon to perform a possible tracheostomy. Safeguarding the patient is the first priority, and time is frequently of the essence.

Change your blade, alter the patient's head position, or have someone else try. Bare in mind, however, that the more laryngoscopies you perform, the more likelihood there is of increasing laryngeal edema or bleeding. This can worsen

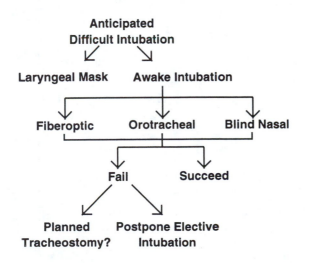

Fig. 11-16. Algorithm for the anticipated difficult intubation.

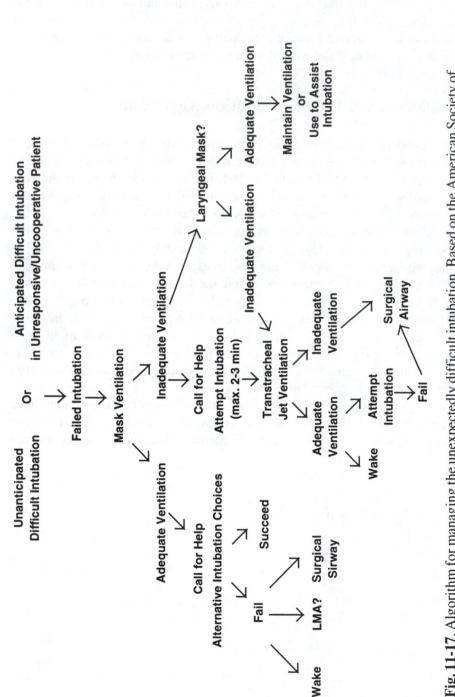

Fig. 11-17. Algorithm for managing the unexpectedly difficult intubation. Based on the American Society of Anesthesiologists Practice Guidelines on Difficult Intubation.

the airway and ultimately make ventilation difficult. Unless you quickly see evidence of impending success, it's better to switch to an alternative method of intubation such as fiberoptic intubation. You can also consider the use of the laryngeal mask airway (LMA) in certain patients. See Chapters 13 and 14 for discussions of the LMA and the fiberoptic.

A more serious situation is the can't intubate/can't ventilate scenario. You have only minutes until life threatening complications will occur, including brain damage and death.

Call for help and for your emergency airway equipment. Try various methods to improve mask ventilation. Try another quick attempt at intubation. Consider the use of a laryngeal mask airway to improve ventilation. If you can wake the patient up, do so. If you can ventilate through the LMA, you may be able to use it as a guide for intubation. This technique is described in Chapter 13.

If ventilation is still poor, place a large bore catheter though the cricothyroid membrane for oxygen administration — optimally by jet ventilator. Once oxygenation is assured limited attempts at intubation can proceed. If these fail, or if you have been unable to establish oxygenation, then a surgical airway is indicated.

See Chapters 13 for discussions of the LMA, jet ventilation, and cricothyrotomy. See Chapter 14 for discussion of fiberoptic intubation. Further information on difficult intubations related to trauma is provided in Chapter 12.

Further Reading

Barrett GE, Coulthard SW: Upper airway obstruction: diagnosis and management options. *Anesthesia and ENT Surgery. Cont. Anesth. Pract.* 1987; 9: 73

Benumof JL. Management of the difficult intubation, with special emphasis on awake adult intubation. *Anes* 1991; 75: 1087-1110

Block C, Brechner VL: Unusual problems in airway management: II The influence of the temporomandibular joint, the mandible, and associated structures in endotracheal intubation. *Anesth. Analg.* 1971; 50: 114

Brechner VL: Unusual problems in airway management: I. Flexion, extension mobility of the cervical vertebrae. *Anesth. Analg.* 1968; 47: 362

Caplan RA, Benumof JL, Berry FA, et al.. Practice guidelines for management of the difficult airway. A report by the Americal Society of Anesthesiologists Task Force on management of the difficult airway. *Anes.* 1993;78: 597-602.

Davies OD: Re-anesthetizing cases of tonsillectomy and adenoidectomy because of persistent postoperative hemorrhage. *Br. J. Anaes.* 1964; 36: 244

Donlon JV: Anesthetic management of the patient with compromised airways. *Anesth. Rev.* 1980; 7: 22

Gordon RA: Anesthetic management of patients with airway problems. *Int. Anesthesiol. Clin.* 1972; 10: 37

12 AIRWAY MANAGEMENT OF TRAUMA

The goals of airway management in trauma are to treat airway obstruction and respiratory insufficiency, avoid aspiration, and improve hemodynamic stability while at the same time taking precautions to protect the spinal cord and brain from further damage.

The presence of trauma complicates airway management in several ways. First, the respiratory system and the airway may be injured with anatomical landmarks distorted or destroyed, making mask ventilation and intubation difficult or impossible.

Second, care of the trauma victim carries with it a degree of uncertainty. The extent or even the nature of the injury isn't always apparent when treatment begins. Deterioration of the patient's condition can occur at any time, requiring careful monitoring and reassessment.

Third, evaluation of multiple injuries can draw attention away from the airway at critical moments.

Airway Evaluation

Interactive Respiratory System

Trauma can injure any component of the respiratory system and impair oxygen transport. Oxygen delivery starts with air passing through the open conduit of the pharynx and the larynx to reach the lungs. Reflex arcs to prevent aspiration must guard the entrance and allow coughing. But the process also depends upon an intact lung alveolar interface with an intact tracheobronchial tree contained within an airtight chest cavity moved by the bellows action of the diaphragm and intercostal muscles. This system is passive and to function requires the medulla of the brain to interpret and react to the peripheral chemical feedback coming in. The control signals from the brain must progress down functioning phrenic and intercostal nerves to drive the bellows. To complete the system, adequate circulatory volume and red blood cells must pass the alveoli to carry oxygen to the periphery. Inefficiency or failure of any component in this complex interactive system requires some form of airway intervention.

This intervention can be as simple as giving supplemental oxygen or as complex as intubating the patient to provide ventilator support.

Airway Assessment

Assessment of the airway takes into account a rapid triage of the urgency of intervention, an initial estimate as to the etiology of the respiratory distress, the state of consiousness of the patient, and the presence or absence of facial trauma.

Carefully assess the patient to decide if the airway status is critical, urgent, or stable. Critical patients need immediate airway intervention to survive. Urgent patients require airway assistance, but there is some time to optimize both the patient and the technique. Even stable patients require continued reassessment.

Respiratory distress in the trauma victim may stem from airway obstruction, pneumothorax, pulmonary contusion, pulmonary aspiration, flail chest, spinal cord injury, and severe shock among other injuries. Rapid assessment of the cause as well as the degree of dysfunction is essential because treatment will vary. For example, placing a chest tube to treat tension pneumothorax may eliminate the respiratory distress and avoid intubation.

Ask conscious victims if they are getting enough air. Their ability to speak to you is a simple but effective screen for the urgency of intervention. Conscious inspiration increases the space in the pharynx and allows better air exchange. Sedation and loss of consciousness cause loss of pharyngeal muscle tone and can collapse this space, worsening obstruction. Giving sedation to any patient with partial airway obstruction carries significant risk of complete airway obstruction and death. If you must sedate then only use light doses of agents such as morphine that are easily reversed. Have the reversal agent at hand. Monitor the patient carefully for worsening obstruction.

Unconscious victims are more difficult to evaluate. Cyanosis is a late sign — often hard to see due to anemia, ambient lighting, and skin color. Examining the airway, listening to the chest, and watching chest wall dynamics are methods that may miss subtle deterioration. Blood gas analysis, and radiologic exam, when available, are reliable, but take time. The loss of protective airway reflexes may go unnoticed   Because of the difficulty, many practitioners routinely intubate the unconscious victim in order to protect the airway and provide improved ventilation to treat possible increased intracranial pressure. When you elect to observe the unconscious victim, you must frequently re-examine him for evidence of respiratory compromise as well as protective airway reflexes. Patients with partial airway obstruction often have noisy breathing, be aware that patients with full airway obstruction often make no noise at all. The absence of stridor in the patient with severe obstruction can be a sign of impending respiratory collapse.

Awake patients with maxillofacial injuries or airway edema often breathe more easily when sitting, flexed forward, and they should be allowed to stay in this position if their other injuries and hemodynamic status permit. A 23% increase in cross-sectional area of the pharynx takes place when the patient moves from supine to sitting (See Reference 1). The sitting position slows further development of edema, lets blood and secretions drain from the mouth, and allows gravity to pull soft tissue forward, out of the airway. Transporting such patients on their side can also minimize airway obstruction when intubation has not been possible.

Airway Management

Establish Air Exchange

The first priority is to establish good air exchange to avoid hypoxia and hypercarbia. The traumatized victim is less likely to be able to tolerate prolonged hypoventilation. Chest wall splinting, altered consciousness, and hemorrhagic anemia, are situations associated with trauma that can result in hypoxemia and hypercarbia.

If the patient obstructs, open the airway while protecting the cervical spine from excessive movement. This often allows adequate gas exchange. Intubation may not be required if the patient rouses sufficiently from relief of hypoxemia. Suction secretions. If available, provide supplemental oxygen. Persistent airway obstruction despite soft tissue manipulation may mean a foreign body is lodged in the airway.

Rarely, intubation may need to precede bag and mask ventilation if the maxillofacial anatomy is destroyed. However, attempt to improve ventilation while the intubation equipment is assembled and checked. Changing the patient's position or pulling forward on the mandible, maxilla, or tongue may open the airway enough to improve gas exchange and buy time.

Risk of Aspiration

Delayed gastric emptying occurs due to pain, shock, ileus, drug effects, CNS injury, and occasionally gastric outlet obstruction. Consider all trauma patients to have full stomachs, regardless of the time or amount of their last meal. Emesis occurs frequently in patients in shock or severe pain. Aspiration of blood, secretions, or stomach contents can occur at any time due to laryngeal incompetence, diminished or absent cough, and altered consciousness — even if emesis does not occur. Awake patients strapped to a back board for transport are helpless if they vomit.

When the trauma patient aspirates, aspiration pneumonitis is likely since the stomach often contains a large volume of particulate matter with low pH. Always be prepared for vomiting by monitoring carefully for oropharyngeal secretions, repetitive swallowing, or retching. Have functioning suction immediately available.

Indications for Intubation

Deciding when to intubate can be difficult. An adequate airway can quickly disappear because of progressive edema, hematoma, or deteriorating hemodynamic status. Clear indications to attempt intubation if possible are:

* full cardiac arrest
* hypovolemic shock with impending arrest
* severe airway obstruction
* unable to ventilate with bag and mask
* deteriorating air exchange with no sign of improvement
* no pharyngeal (gag) reflexes
* head injury with a Glascow coma scale less than 7–8 (see Table 12-1)

Table 12–1. Glascow Coma Score.

Eye Opening (E)	
Spontaneous	4
To Speech	3
To pain	2
None	1
Best Motor Response (M)	
Obeys	6
Localizes	5
Withdraws	4
Abnormal flexion	3
Abnormal extention	2
None	1
Verbal (V)	
Oriented	5
Confused conversation	4
Inappropriate words	3
Incomprehensible words	2
None	1
Coma Score = E + M + V (ie. 3 to 15)	

- potential for increased intracranial pressure with hypoventilation.

The preceding situations are those where the patient is unable to adequately ventilate, is unable to protect the airway from aspiration, or must receive hyperventilation to decrease incranial pressure.

Marked airway obstruction is an obvious indication to assist the patient with a mask and then intubate. The common signs of airway obstruction are:

- inspiratory stridor
- rocking chest motion

  chest falls on inspiration/abdomen rises on inspiration
- use of accessory muscles of respiration
- tracheal tug
- faint or absent breath sounds
- poor movement of air
- cyanosis

(See Chapter 3 for further explanation.)

Unfortunately, especially in the trauma victim, indications are not always clear. Decisions must often be made before a clear picture of obstruction presents. Symptoms and signs of increasing airway obstruction may be subtle and occasionally one must have a high index of suspicion to indentify them. The common signs of airway decompensation are:

- inability to swallow, drooling
- *expiratory* snore or fluttering sound — *may* indicate increasing edema
- altered voice: hoarseness, weakness, "strangled" voice
- persistent and severe sore throat
- intermittent obstruction
- symptoms worsen with forced ventilation
- inability to make a high pitched "e" sound
- *restlessness or disorientation may mean hypoxia and hypercarbia*

The decision to intubate in the face of such subtle signs is a judgment call and should be based on proximity to the hospital if in the field, concurrent injuries, progression of symptoms, if any, the mechanism of injury, and the skill and available equipment of the caregiver. Ask yourself what will happen if you do nothing? If you decide to wait, observe the patient carefully, reassess often, and place him as quickly as possible into a hospital setting where continued evaluation and possibly intubation can take place if needed.

Intubation Technique: Protecting the Cervical Spine

Any intubation technique must take the potential for cervical spine (CS) injury into account. A review article by Hastings and Marks (2) provides an excellent summary of the risks of CS injury (Table 12-2).

Since even minor trauma may injure the cervical spine (CS) it is imperativ e that the head and neck be stabilized to avoid excessive extension, flexion, or distraction until injury is ruled out. If you think CS injury is possible you should use stabilization methods. Soft cervical collars allow 75% of normal movement, rigid collars allow about 30% flexion/extension and 50% lateral turning. The best method, securing the victim from head to foot on a backboard, with further stabilization of the neck with sandbags and a rigid collar allows only 5% of normal movement (3).

Longstanding controversy exists as to the best method of securing the airway in the presence of possible cervial spine injury. Three options for intubation exist: nasal intubation, oral intubation, or surgical airway. The technique chosen for intubation depends on:

- urgency
- need for cervical spine immobilization and protection
- aspiration prevention
- severity of airway compromise
- potential for difficult intubation (i.e. "anterior airway," facial trauma)

Table 12-2. Risk of Cervical Spine Injury.

Known Injury
      Positive C-Spine Xrays or CT scan
      Neurologic Deficit
High-Risk (>10%)

      Front-end MVA > 35 mph without seatbelt
      Head-first fall
      Equivocal C-spine Xray
Moderate Risk (1–2%)

      MVA
      Head injury
      Non-head first fall
      Contact sport injury
      High-risk group with negative C-spine Xrays
No-Risk
      Alert patient without neck pain or tenderness
      Negative C-spine Xrays (3 views)
      Negative C-spine CT scan

- associated medical conditions (i.e. angina, head injury, shock)
- conscious or unconscious patient
- cooperative or uncooperative patient
- intubator's expertise with the different techniques

Awake nasal intubation is frequently recommended in the patient with potential CS injury as a means of avoiding neurologic damage. However, nasal intubation in the trauma victim has several disadvantages.

The risk of cannulating the brain contraindicates its use in nasal, midface, or basilar skull fractures because of possible associated cribiform plate fracture. Severe nose bleeds can occur in dilutional coagulopathies, seen in many trauma victims. Tube manipulations in the posterior pharynx may cause retching — which can worsen ICP, bronchospasm, and cause laryngospasm. In addition, inability to manipulate the head and neck to protect the CS may lead to a prolonged intubation attempt that a hypoxemic patient can ill afford.

Blind nasal intubation is difficult in frightened, drunk, obtunded, or combative patients, and in children. More than 50% of trauma victims are under the influence of drugs or alcohol. One study performed by emergency medicine physicians comparing safety and efficacy of nasal vs. oral intubations in intoxicated patients showed that oral intubation was preferable. In their study, it had a higher success rate (100% oral vs 65% nasal), was faster, required fewer attempts, and had fewer complications (0% oral, 69% nasal)(4). However, it should be noted that they used the muscle relaxant succinylcholine when necessary, a technique which also carries potential hazards to be discussed later.

Prolonged nasal intubations can lead to sinusitis and sepsis.

Finally, in many areas of the country, paramedics and nurse responders are not certified for nasal intubation. In these areas, patients are intubated in the field orally or not at all. Carefully performing a necessary oral intubation is better than not intubating someone who needs it and cannot receive adequate ventilation by other means.

In the critical patient, direct laryngoscopy is the fastest and surest method of intubating, but it does requires some atlanto-occipital extention, even if the CS is immobilized. While slightly more motion of the cervical spine takes place with oral as opposed to careful nasal intubation, it has yet to be documented that this fracture movement damages the spinal cord (5,6,7,8). The Cervical Spine Research Society reported a neurologic complication rate of 1% in 5,356 major cervical procedures. Increasing data support the careful use of oral tracheal intubation and muscle relaxants in the CS injured patient, although there is a need to proceed with caution. When immediate airway intervention is not necessary, awake techniques and fiberoptic intubation should be considered. In the stable patient, definitive work-up to evaluate potential CS injury should occur and if present the patient should be immobilized as indicated.

Careful oral intubation of critical patients using manual in-line axial "traction," or MIAT, is a feasible alternative to nasal intubation (5). Traction is probably not the best word, since the goal of MIAT is to stabilize the spine and prevent further injury. The assistant stabilizing the neck must balance the need for static immobilization versus active traction, a task which is not easy. Use your neurosurgeon if he or she is immediately available. However, in the absence of a neurosurgeon have your assistant grip the head at the mastoid processes bilaterally and hold it in a neutral position without pulling on the head. (see Fig. 11-15, pg. 138.) You can also have your assistant pull on the hair to stabilize the head. Remove any obstructions to the mouth such as cervical collars prior to attempting oral intubation. Cricoid pressure — if used — must be gentle.

Stabilizing the patient's head and neck can be awkward when the patient is on the ground. While an assistant can use the MIAT technique, it's difficult for him to stay out of the intubator's way. It's often easier for the intubator to provide her own stabilization by placing the head and neck between her own knees (see Fig. 12–1). Leaning backward provides the distance needed to manipulate the tube and visualize the larynx.

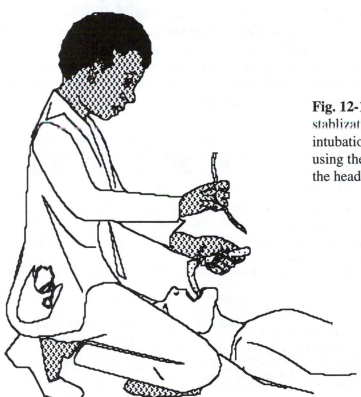

Fig. 12-1. Cervical stablization during intubation on the ground using the knees to hold the head.

Cricoid pressure frequently helps visualization as well as guards against aspiration. However, use this technique with caution in patients with suspected laryngeal or cervical spine injuries and don't hesitate to omit it if you feel it's contraindicated.

The Laryngeal Mask Airway or LMA can also be used both to provide ventilation and to assist intubation when intubation has proved difficult. The LMA should not be a first choice for airway management in trauma victims because these patients are at high risk for vomiting. The LMA does not protect against aspiration. The LMA is a good adjunct when oropharyngeal anatomy is undamaged and no fixed obstruction exists above the glottis. The LMA is a poorer choice when the anatomy has been distorted by trauma or edema or if fixed upper airway obstruction exists. These latter situations might prevent a good seal and interfere with ventilation. You can also secure the airway with a Combitube™. Both of these devices are described in Chapter 13.

Fiberoptic laryngoscopy can be used to assist both nasal and oral intubations. It's use in trauma is often hampered by its lack of availability in the field, lack of familiarity with the instrument, blood in the oropharynx, distortion of the anatomy, edema, combative patients, and the need for speed in the presence of hypoxemia. Intubators need to practice extensively with the instrument prior to using it in trauma victims.

Trauma victims, with often marginal oxygenation, cannot tolerate prolonged, repetitive attempts at intubation. Make sure you provide supplementary oxygen and suction the airway as needed during your attempts. Have a low threshold for proceeding to a surgical airway if your initial attempts fail and the patient's airway status is critical, especially if the anatomy is destroyed by trauma.

Potential indications for a surgical airway are:

- combined bilateral mandibular fractures and Le Forte maxillary fractures
- gross deformity, edema of oropharynx or tongue
- gunshot wounds to the face
- extensive facial burns or crush injury
- cervical spine injury
- penetrating injury to the neck

The techniques for surgical airway are described elsewhere in the text.

Intubating with a Field Airway in Place

If the patient has an esophageal obturator airway and requires intubation, place the endotracheal tube prior to removing the obturator to avoid aspiration. After verifying endotracheal tube placement, deflate the obturator cuff and remove it. Be prepared for vomiting. (See Chapter 13.)

Don't forget the rest of the patient

It's very easy in the urgency of establishing an airway to forget about the rest of the patient. Hemodynamic changes associated with intubation can lead to further decompensation of the rest of the patient's medical problems. Check blood pressure, pulse, and oxygen saturation frequently if available.

Similarly, urgent control of hemorrhage, placement of intravenous access and chest tubes, and ongoing diagnosis of the extent and nature of the patient's injuries can allow the team to lose sight of progressive airway obstruction.

Don't become fixated on one aspect of the patient's care.

Adjuncts to Intubation

Use of Sedatives and Local Anesthetics

The advantages and disadvantages of the use of sedatives and local anesthetics are discussed in detail in Chapters 15 and 16. Any sedative can cause hypotension when only circulating catecholamines are maintaining the blood pressure. Add sedatives slowly and give them time to work before adding more. Individualize treatment. Small increments of sedation and topical anesthesia may be all you need to control the unruly patient. However, the line between sedation and apnea is sometimes quite slim, especially in the presence of hypoxia or hypotension.

Don't use *injected* local anesthetic blocks in patients who are fighting. You can't guarantee against intravascular injection of the drug. In these patients topical cetacaine or lidocaine spray work well. Lidocaine ointment or gel down the nose can help make nasal intubation tolerable. Never leave the patient alone once you start to topicalize the airway and have suction ready to use. Even if the trachea itself is not anesthetized, other protective airway reflexes have been altered. It takes several minutes for local anesthesia to numb the mucous membranes and it's often impossible to wait in an emergency.

Avoid numbing below the vocal cords until after the tube is placed to allow some protection against aspiration. However, spraying intravenous li-docaine (50–100mg) down the endotracheal tube after intubation often allows semiconscious patients to tolerate the tube better. Intra-tracheal lidocaine is rapidly absorbed systemically — be careful to consider the total dosage of topical lidocaine given in your toxic dose calculations.

Use of Muscle Relaxants and Induction Agents

Muscle relaxants are medications which produce temporary paralysis of all the patient's muscles. They are commonly used in combination with general anesthetic induction agents during surgery to allow rapid intubation as well as to produce a relaxed field for the surgeon to expedite the operation. Muscle relaxants do not themselves produce loss of consciousness or amnesia. Their use to intubate trauma patients in the field or in the emergency room is controversial and must be individualized to the patient. Muscle relaxants combined with an agent to induce unconsciousness can facilitate intubation in the patient who struggles, which can decrease intubation trauma. Faster intubations often cause fewer physiologic changes and can allow faster treatment of hypoxia, hypercarbia, or aspiration risk. Muscle relaxants should *not* be used when bag and mask ventilation cannot be ensured. See Chapter 16 for a more detailed discussion.

Special Considerations

Problems in the Field

Paramedics, nurses, and physicians working at the accident site face multiple problems that hospital care-givers never experience. First, the healthcare worker in the field may face personal injury from vehicles, fire, toxic exposure, and smoke. Distractions abound. An audience of sobbing family members makes dispassionate assessment difficult at best. Care under these circumstances produces more anxiety than caring for the same patient in the emergency room. Even the healthcare worker accustomed to the sight of blood and trauma may be emotionally repelled by the severity of injury — especially in young, previously healthy individuals.

Multiple trauma victims may force prioritizing of treatment to take place. Salvageable patients with inadequate respiration must receive immediate care to prevent irreversible hypoxemia and death.

Noise and sirens drown out breath sounds and heart sounds. Nighttime lighting, head lights, and flashing red strobes hide cyanosis and pallor. Daylight has a bluer cast than indoor tungsten lighting and makes skin color harder to judge. Even feeling a pulse in a vibrating ambulance or helicopter may prove impossible.

Because assessment at the scene is more difficult, the caregiver must be more attentive to the potential for subtle or delayed signs of respiratory embarrassment. Use *all* the senses. If you can't hear breath sounds because of noise then feel for movement of air out of the nose and mouth with your hand. If you can't see the chest rise, place your hand on the chest to feel it rise in conjunction with air movement. Shining your flashlight on the eye's conjunctiva or inside the mouth may pick up cyanosis when skin color is ambiguous. Placing your ear near the mouth may allow you to pick up stridor that you otherwise can't hear.

Intubation in the field is technically harder. Patients may be trapped in awkward and precarious situations. Nasal intubation in the spontaneously breathing patient is usually easiest in these situations. But in the face of facial or basilar skull fractures, or when a paramedic or nurse is not certified to perform nasal intubations, the need for oral intubations may arise. Orally intubating a patient pinned in a sitting position behind the steering wheel of his car is certainly difficult, but can often be successfully done. Barring anatomical distortion from edema or direct trauma, the anatomy of the airway does not change when the patient's position changes. If you have access to the airway and room to maneuver you can orally intubate in unusual positions.

Practice with a mannikin in sitting, lateral, and prone positions to familiarize yourself with the problems of visualizing the anatomy, stabilizing the head, and positioning yourself for best mechanical advantage. Mental rehearsal and practice for difficult situations helps greatly when facing the unknown. If you believe that it's possible to intubate under these cir–cumstances you'll frequently prove yourself correct.

Most paramedic protocols allow three intubation attempts in the field before aborting the procedure. If intubation fails, use nasal or oral airways, mask assistance, and patient positioning to optimize ventilation during transport. Grasping the tongue or mandible with a clamp or suture and pulling it forward can help in mandibular fractures and massive tongue edema. Pulling the maxilla forward can open the airway in patient's with midface fractures. Use an endotracheal tube adapter to attach a nasal airway to the ambu bag and ventilate by closing the patient's mouth and opposite nostril   (see Fig. 3-4, pg. 48). Suction frequently as needed.

Noise, distractions, anxiety, and awkward positioning make inadvertant eso–phageal intubation more likely, and more difficult to recognize. Moving the patient repetitively from site of injury to stretcher, to ambulance, to hospital means extubation can occur at any time. Reassess the correct positioning of the endotracheal tube **every time** you move the patient, regardless of how minor the repositioning. If the respiratory status deteriorates check the position of the tube in addition to ruling out pneumothorax, etc. Always have a high index of suspicion for extubation and esophageal intubation.

Listen to your co-workers. If someone suggests that you are not ventilating well, or that the endotracheal tube may be esophageal don't become defensive. Instead, check the patient and verify the location of the endotracheal tube. It's better to perform an unnecessary check than it is to miss a problem because of pride.

Blood in the Oropharynx

Blood in the oropharynx predisposes the patient to aspiration and hypoxia. In the worst case scenario, the patient is unconscious, unable to protect their airway, and is bleeding so badly that you can't see any landmarks at all. It's a frightening experience.

The patient needs ventilation and oxygen. If they are breathing well on their own give them supplemental oxygen, start intravenous volume replacement, and supply suction for the airway. Ventilate them if they are not breathing adequately. Place these patients in a position that allows the blood to drain away from the airway. For example, place them on their side or sitting up leaning forward. Never let them lay face up and flat. If they must be supine, as during CPR, then place the bed in Trendelenburg to allow the blood to pool in the upper pharynx, away from the airway. Suction the mouth frequently. You may need to keep a soft suction cather or the main suction tubing itself in the mouth to suction continuously. Turn the face to the side if you can. If you hear gurgling as the patient ventilates, then suction the patient. Patients who can't protect their airways need intubation as quickly as possible.

You can manually ventilate patients on their side, if spinal precautions are not needed. You may need help maintaining the mask seal. Have someone check breath sounds. It is far easier to place the patient left side down. This way the left hand can hold the mask while resting on the bed and the right one can ventilate freely. Right side down points the bag into the bed, forcing you to reverse the equipment (Fig. 12-2a, b).

If the bleeding is serious, you may prefer to intubate the patient on her side (Fig. 12-3). Again, left side down is optimal. Your left hand pushes the tongue to the left during laryngoscopy. With the left side down, gravity helps pull the tongue out of the way. It also leaves plenty of room for your right arm to maneuver the tube. The anatomy is the same and you should not let the different position unnerve you. You won't have the weight of the head pulling it down during laryngoscopy because the head stays on the bed. The blade may pull the head without lifting the jaw. If this is a problem, have a helper hold the head steady as you look.

Inexperienced and experienced intubators alike may prefer a combined method. Place the patient left side down and in slight Trendelenburg to ventilate the patient until everything is ready for intubation. Use cricoid pressure to prevent passive regurgitation of swallowed blood and secretions. Cricoid pressure may not prevent aspiration of the blood pooling in the oropharynx so suction frequently as you wait. Just before intubation clean the airway thoroughly, hand the suction catheter to an assistant, and turn the patient onto his back. Maintain cricoid pressure. Intubate him quickly. Have your assistant suction the airway as you work if needed.

If your first attempt fails use your judgement about turning the patient lateral or keeping him supine. Whichever you choose, suction the airway well between attempts. When the anatomy is covered in blood, identification of landmarks can be difficult. Look for air bubbles coming from the larynx as a clue to the location of the cords. A gentle, abrupt push on the chest by an assistant can provide bubbles for you if the patient isn't breathing. If the patient is breathing, you will hear breath sounds through the endotracheal tube. These sounds will stop instantly if the tube enters the esophagus. Use the breath sounds as another clue to tube position.

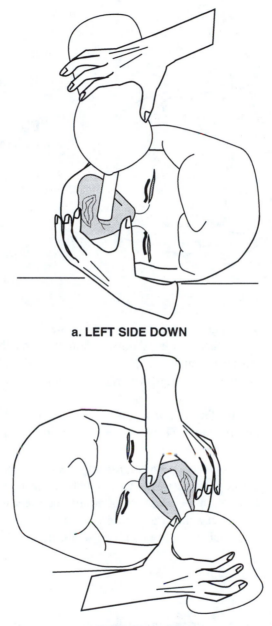

a. LEFT SIDE DOWN

b. RIGHT SIDE DOWN

Fig. 12-2. Ventilating the patient on his side. Ventilation with left side down is easiest. The hand squeezing the bag is free to move, with the right side down, the angle of your hands is awkward and the bag bumps into the bed.

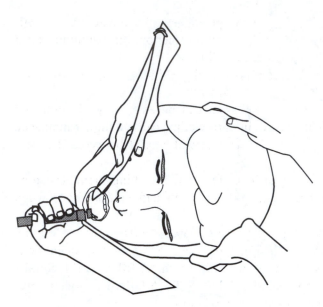

Fig. 12-3. Intubation with the head left side down. Notice helper stabilizing head.

After intubating, thoroughly suction the endotracheal tube as aspiration of blood is very common in these cases. Another danger is that blood left in the tube may clot, obstructing the tube and preventing ventilation. These clots can become so solid that the tube must be removed and replaced, sometimes emergently.

If the source of the bleeding is **above** the glottis, such as nosebleed, the patient is unconsious, and the situation is critical. Placement of an LMA may secure the airway and provide some minimum of airway protection. The LMA may then be used to facilitate intubation, either as a direct conduit or by using the fiberoptic bronchoscope. The LMA would help to provide a clear visual field for the fiberoptic, even in the presence of continued bleeding.

An LMA does not protect against aspiration of gastric contents. The patient with bleeding into the oropharynx is at high risk due to swallowed blood. Be prepared for vomiting.

You can also use a Combitube™ to secure the airway.

Burn Victims

Airway obstuction can occur precipitously in the burn victim. The patient is at high risk if the injury occured in an enclosed space or involved steam, especially with prolonged exposure. Examine the victim for facial burns, singed nasal hair, carbonaceous material in the nose or oropharynx. Look in the mouth for blisters on the hard palate, redness or marked inflammation of the oropharynx, and red/dry mucosa. Does the victim complain of hoarseness, dyspnea, or sore throat? Is there carbonaceous sputum or a cough? The combination of any of these in a high risk patient causes many physicians to intubate prophylactically, rather than waiting for evidence if airway obstruction. Fifteen minutes can make a huge difference in oropharyngeal swelling.

The patient can still be at risk even if none of these signs and symptoms is initially present and should be re-evaluated frequently.

Once airway obstruction occurs, intubation can be extremely difficult and sometimes inpossible. Surgical airways in burn victims cause a higher incidence of complications and mortality than intubation, and should be avoided unless absolutely necessary.

Provide a high FiO_2. The four-hour half-life of CO breathing room air can be reduced to one hour when breathing 100% oxygen and half an hour when breathing hyperbaric oxygen.

Burn victims may also suffer respiratory collapse, independent of airway problems, due to toxic fumes such as CO, hydrogen cyanide, and nitrogen dioxide, among other products of combustion in our synthetic filled world. Smoke inhalation can also lead to pneumonias and ARDS. Such failure can occur anytime during the first several days following the injury.

Severe Facial Injuries

Always assume that the patient with severe facial injuries has a possible cervical spine injury or the potential for head injury and take appropriate precautions. If the patient has adequate respirations you have time to rule out concurrent injuries. Be aware, however, that such injuries are often dynamic and severe airway obstruction can occur at any time. Bleeding or edema formation within the retropharyngeal planes can cause abrupt worsening of the airway. Foreign bodies in the form of bone fragments and tissue may cause abrupt airway obstruction. There is little relationship between the external findings and the severity of skeletal injuries — it's often better to err on the side of early intubation than to wait for the development of complications at a later, less controlled time.

Midface fractures allowing the maxilla to fall into the airway can cause obstruction. The mandible is often pulled backwards by the strong facial muscles in patients with bimandibular fractures. Orally intubating such a patient risks damage to nerves as the fracture shifts.

Blind nasal intubation is relatively contraindicated due to potential cribiform plate rupture and the risk for passing the endotracheal tube or fracture material into the cranial vault or the brain itself. If the need to proceed to intubation is critical and X-rays are not available, a quick exam of the nasal passages with a gloved and lubricated finger can establish whether the passage appears intact. When in doubt use an alternate technique.

Oral intubation may be possible even in the presence of severe facial trauma. You should consider proceeding to a surgical airway in a patient with destroyed anatomy if you have any difficulty providing adequate ventilation.

The patient may be unable to open his mouth for several reasons. Trismus, or masseter spasm, is very common in facial fractures and will respond to the administration of an anesthetic and muscle relaxant (see Chapter 16). On the other hand, temporomandibular joint dysfunction due to injury of the joint itself can also lock the jaw shut and this will not respond to muscle relaxants. You will not be able to distinguish between the two entities acutely without radiologic exam. Awake intubation is recommended for these cases until the pathology is known. Trismus lasting longer than two weeks may cause permanent fibrosis and partial freezing of the joint.

Head Injury

Patients presenting with altered mental status may or may not have obvious signs of head injury such as scalp lacerations, postauricular ecchymosis ("Battles" sign,) bilateral black eyes ("racoon eyes"), unequal pupils, or blood behind the eardrum. Any patient with possible head injury should be treated as though they have the potential for increased intracranial pressure (ICP) because even a short noxious stimulus such as laryngoscopy can elevate the ICP for prolonged periods. This can lead to increasing cerebral edema, compromising blood flow, and potentially herniating the brain.

Heavy sedation, topicalization of the airway, and muscle relaxants can allow rapid control of the airway with minimal stimulation or increase in ICP. In addition, lidocaine, pentothal, and etomidate can directly decrease ICP by causing cerebral vasoconstriction. However, one must weigh the benefits of prophylactic ICP treatment against the potential complications such as shock or airway obstruction. Ketamine can raise ICP and increase cerebral metabolism and should be avoided.

Hyperventilate head-injured patients vigorously both before and after intubation to lower pCO_2. Hypocarbia causes cerebral vasoconstriction and thereby decreases ICP. Hyperventilation also helps treat any hypoxemia. Lidocaine 50–100 mg down the endotracheal tube can improve tolerance of the tube and avoid increased ICP due to coughing.

Laryngeal Trauma

Laryngotracheal injury is suggested by the following non-specific signs after blunt or penetrating neck trauma:

- hoarseness
- dyspnea
- painful swallowing
- cervical ecchymosis or swelling
- absence of thyroid prominence
- muffled voice
- difficulty swallowing
- cervical pain and tenderness
- subcutaneous emphysema
- hemoptysis

Patients with suspected laryngeal trauma should be carefully examinined with direct and indirect layngoscopy, soft tissue neck X-rays, endoscopy, and possibly CT scan if time permits. However, respiratory distress requires immediate intubation or, if this fails tracheostomy.

Recommendations for airway control differ. In controlled situations in which the patient has an adequate airway, the anatomical derrangement is known, and the intubator is experienced, then careful direct laryngoscopy may be tried. However, using a fiberoptic bronchoscope is prudent to directly visualize infraglottic structures. You can expedite intubation by combining the techniques, using laryngoscopy to identify the larynx, then using the fiberoptic to visualize the trachea prior to advancing the tube.

Have the equipment and personnel immediately available for performing a surgical airway. Blind techniques can potentially complete a partial laryngotracheal disruption and should be avoided if there is any question of laryngeal injury. In severe airway obstruction proceed directly to tracheostomy. Cricothyroidotomy is contraindicated in the presence of blunt laryngotracheal trauma because of the possibility of acute cricotracheal separation or the creation of a false passage.

Laryngotracheal trauma frequently isn't recognized during intial stabilization and intubation. Conventional intubation, without special precautions, carries the risk of precipitating airway obstruction. Have a high index of suspicion in the presence of head and neck trauma. Signs include difficulty advancing the tube or the tube tip appearing as a bulging mass in the anterior neck suggesting a false passage.

Traumatic rupture of the trachea and bronchi may produce few inital signs and symptoms if the leak is small. This injury is more likely to occur with "clothesline" or handlebar injuries to the neck. These patients are frequently intubated by the time increasing pneumothorax, persistant air leak, and subcutaneous emphysema reveal the injury. If rupture is known prior to intubation, a sterile, single or double lumen tube can be carefully passed — preferably into the uninjured bronchus. Position the cuff **below** the site of injury. Don't force the tube if you feel any resistance at all. A fiberoptic bronchoscope can be used as a stent to position the tube and minimize the risk of complete tracheobroncheal disruption.

Pediatric Patients

Pediatric patients are more prone to airway obstruction and respiratory failure than adults (see Chapter 9) and must be closely observed. Special care must be taken to minimize further insult to their airway. Although awake nasal or oral intubations are common in the adult, these techniques are physically and psychologically traumatic in the infant and small child. They can exacerbate edema and bleeding in an already marginal airway and should be avoided unless absolutely necessary. Intubation is preferable to a surgical airway in the infant or child because tracheostomy is difficult, even in experienced surgical hands.

The incidence of CS trauma is lower in infants (0.5%) and increases with the age of the child and the violence of the accident. It also tends to be higher, at the C1,2 level due to the more horizontal facet joints and laxer ligaments at these levels (9,10). Thus when intubation is performed in a high risk victim great care should be taken to stabilize the cervical spine.

Stress and the Caregiver

Early therapeutic intervention improves patient outcome and survival. This puts pressure on caregivers to make rapid decisions, often before all the facts are known. For example, the decision to intubate a minimally symptomatic burn victim is a judgement call which may avoid the potential need for a later emergent tracheostomy — a technique which in burn victims carries a high risk of mortality from infection.

Awkward positioning of trapped victims and the risk of injury to rescuers themselves complicate care at the scene of the accident. Trauma scenes where the caregiver must triage multiple victims and decide who gets care and who does not, can leave the caregiver guilt ridden even for a job well done.

The severity of trauma injuries, the need to face the acute grief of a patient's family, and the reminder of one's own mortality, make care of the trauma victim much more emotionally draining for the caregiver than other types of patients.

Unfortunately it is also true that a patient can develop serious complications or die even if you make all the correct decisions. When dealing with trauma you must do the best you can with what you have and realize that sometimes even your best isn't good enough.

Every caregiver faces these difficult emotions and should not face them alone. Sharing your feelings and distress with others can make you a better provider and will help prevent burnout.

References

1. American College of Surgeon's Committee on Trauma. *Advanced Trauma Life Support Course, Instructor Manual.* Chicago:American College of Surgeons1984:157–160.

2. Hastings RH, Marks JD: Airway Management for Trauma Patients with Potential Cervical Spine Injuries. *Anesth Analg* 73:471–82, 1991.

3. Podolsky S, Baraff L, et al: Efficacy of Cervical Spine Immobilization Methods. *J Trauma* 23: 461–5, 1983.

4. Majernick TG, Bierniek R, Houston JB, et al: Cervical Spine Movement During Orotracheal Intubation. *Ann Emerg Med* 15:417–420. 1986.

5. Grande CM, Stene JK, Bernhard WN: Airway Management: Considerations in the Trauma Patient. *Crit Care Clin* Vol 6, No.1: 37–59, 1990.

6. Donen SC, Merigan KS, Hedges JR, et al: A comparison of blind nasotracheal and succinylcholine assistant intubation in the poisoned patient. *Ann Emerg Med* 16:75—77, 1987.

7. Wright SW, Robinson GG, Wright MB: Cervical Spine Injuries in Blunt Trauma Patients Requireing Emergent Endotracheal Intubation. *Am J Emerg Med* 10:104–109, 1992

8. Suderman VS, Crosby ET, Lui A: Elective Oral Tracheal Intubation in Cervical Spine Injured Adults. *Can J Anaesth* 38: 785–789, 1991.

9. Bohn D, Armstrong D, Becker L, Humphreys R: Cervical Spine Injuries in Children. *J Trauma* 30:463–9, 1990.

10. Fesmire F, Luten R. The Pediatric Cervical Spine: Developmental Anatomy and clinical Aspects. *J Emerg Med* 7:133–42, 1989.

13   SPECIALIZED VENTILATION TECHNIQUES

The Esophageal Obturator Airway (EOA), the Esophageal-Tracheal Combitube, and the Laryngeal Mask Airway (LMA) are specialized devices for ventilating the patient without intubation. These devices are often used in emergency situations when intubation cannot be performed and mask ventilation is felt to be inadequate airway protection.

Needle and surgical cricothyroidotomy are useful emergency techniques for oxygenating and establishing an airway.

Esophageal Obturator Airway

The EOA is only used in the field as an alternative to bag and mask ventilation. It does not provide better ventilation than any other properly used bag-valve-mask device. The airway must be maintained open in the same way. The EOA does provide a barrier to minimize regurgitation of gastric contents. The use of the EOA carries risks of patient injury and death if used incorrectly or in a rough fashion. It should not be considered a replacement to intubation, merely an interim form of airway management until intubation can occur.

The EOA consists of a long tube — open at the top and sealed at the bottom — with multiple small holes near the upper end. A special mask fits over the tube and seals against the patient's face in the usual manner. The ventilation bag is then attached to the tube as it exits the top of the mask. The large cuff on the EOA is designed to seal the esophagus, thereby preventing regurgitation and preventing air from entering the stomach.

Insertion of the EOA
To assemble the EOA, place its top through the port in the mask. Check the cuff by inflation with 20–30 cc of air. Deflate the cuff prior to insertion. Lubricate the end with water soluble jelly.

To insert the EOA flex the head slightly and pull the jaw forward (Fig. 13–1). Gently advance the tube down the patient's throat into the esophagus until the mask sits against the face. Never force the tube. If there is resistence pull back and readvance. Try gently twisting it.

Once in position you must check the location of the EOA *before* inflating the cuff. This is different than endotracheal intubation. Correct placement of the EOA in the esophagus will allow you to ventilate the patient. Incorrect placement of the EOA into the trachea will prevent all ventilation because the end of the EOA is closed. Inflation of the large EOA cuff if misplaced in the trachea can lead to tracheal rupture as well as asphyxia if the error is not recognized. If the EOA is in the trachea remove it immediately and ventilate the patient by mask prior to the next attempt.

Cautions in the Use of the EOA

- The EOA should be used only in the deeply unconsious patient because it will cause gagging and vomiting in the awake or semiconsious patient.
- Don't use it in children under 16 years old or under 5 ft. tall.
- Don't use the EOA in patients with known esophageal disease such as varices or ingestion of a caustic substance.

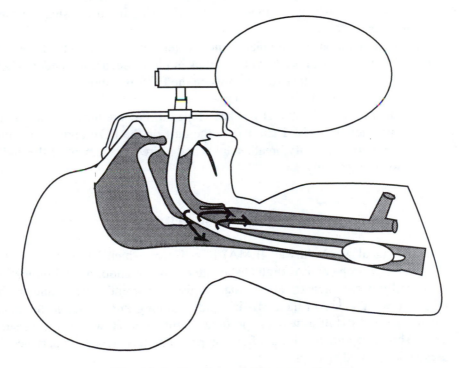

Fig. 13-1. Esophageal Obturator Airway

- The EOA cannot be suctioned and therefore allows the build up of gastric contents and pressure during use. Never remove the EOA from an unconsious patient until the patient has been intubated. Vomiting and aspiration could occur.

- Asphyxia and death can occur if the EOA is postioned in the trachea.

At least one paramedic study has compared the incidence of complications of the EOA to intubation (1). In a review of 509 consecutive cardiac arrests treated, EOA placement was successful in 86.7% while only 66.9% of the intubations were successful on first attempt and an additional 30% successful on second attempt. However, the complication rate for the EOA was higher, 11.1% vs 7.7%. Complications for the EOA included misplacement, kinking, curling, swelling/hematoma, and traumatic extubation. Those for intubation included extubation and misplacement. Fatalities were markedly different, with EOA complications 8.7% fatal compared to 2.6% for intubation. The EOA must be used with caution in the field.

Intubation with the EOA in Place

Prepare your equipment and hyperventilate the patient prior to the attempt. You won't be able to ventilate the patient with the mask removed. To remove the mask, pinch the EOA near the port and slide it off. Push the EOA as far to the left of the mouth as you can to get it out of the way. Intubate using the standard techniques.

Once the intubation is complete immediately verify correct placement. Esophageal intubation can occur with an EOA in place. Secure the endotracheal tube well to avoid accidental extubation when the EOA is removed.

To remove the EOA have an assistant hold the endotracheal tube firmly in place no matter how well you feel you have taped it. Prepare for possible vomiting by having suction ready. Then deflate the cuff on the EOA and gently slide it out of the mouth. Reverify breath sounds and correct placement of the endotracheal tube immediately.

Laryngeal Mask Airway

The Laryngeal Mask Airway (LMA) is a device which has been used for many years in Europe and Australia as an alternative to endotracheal intubation for selected types of general anesthesia. Its use is currently increasing in the United States. The use of the LMA is rapidly gaining importance in the management of the difficult airway or the failed intubation. However, use in such patients should optimally occur after the provider has gained experience in patients with normal airways.

The LMA looks like a short endotracheal tube with a small cushioned mask on its distal end (Fig. 13–2). It was designed using the pharynx of the adult cadaver as a model. When in use, the balloon cushion on the mask is inflated once the mask overlies the laryngeal outlet, sealing that space and allowing positive pressure ventilation. The opening in the mask is covered by a soft, flexible grill which helps prevent entrapment of the epiglottis in the mask opening. It also helps prevent obstruction of the opening by the epiglottis if it folds over the larynx.

When perfectly positioned, the cushion lies with its tip against the upper esophageal sphincter. The sides face the piriform sinuses with the upper surface behind the base of the tongue and the epiglottis pointing upwards. This ideal positioning happens about 50-60% of the time. When the epiglottis is within the rim of the LMA, it is folded downward 50-90% of the time and the lateral aryepiglottic folds are folded inward 50% of the time. Although the actual position of the LMA often varies from the ideal, ventilation is rarely impaired and is judged without difficulty in 95-99% of patients in most studies.

The LMA is inserted blindly, without the use of a laryngoscope. It has been successfully used in emergency situations where intubation has proved impossible. It's also easy for the inexperienced provider to use. One study of paramedical and medical students showed that 94% of the students successfully ventilated the patient on the first try using the LMA while only 69% succeeded in endotracheally intubating the patient on their first try.

Insertion Technique

Choose the correct size mask (Table 13–1).

Prior to placing the LMA, inflate the cushion on the mask and check for leaks or abnormal bulging. Then deflate the cushion with the cushion gently pressed against a flat surface (Fig. 13-3). This allows the cushion to be wrinkle free. Make sure that the rim curves upward, away from the opening.

It's crucial that the leading edge of the cuff be smooth and wrinkle free. This helps prevent the tip of the deflated cushion from curling, a shape which could potentially fold the epiglottis down over the glottis during insertion, or prevent a good seal (Fig. 13-4).

Lubricate the posterior surface of the LMA. Never lubricate the anterior surface, where the grill is, because lubricant can obstruct the opening or trickle down the larynx.

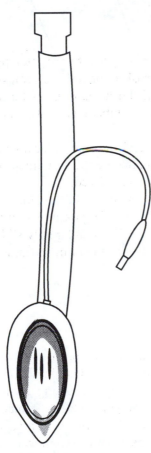

Fig. 13-2. Laryngeal Mask Airway.

Table 13–1. Laryngeal Mask Sizes.

Size 1:	Neonates/infants up to 6.5 kg
Size 2:	Infants and children up to 20 kg
Size 2.5:	Children 20–30 kg
Size 3:	Children and small adults over 30 kg
Size 4:	Normal and large adults
Size 5:	Extra large adults

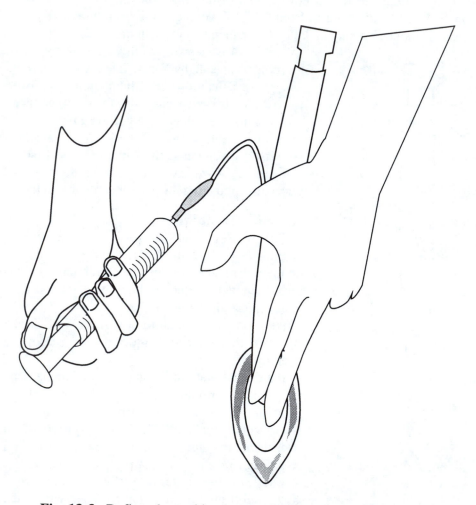

Fig. 13-3. Deflate the cushion by pressing it against a flat surface.

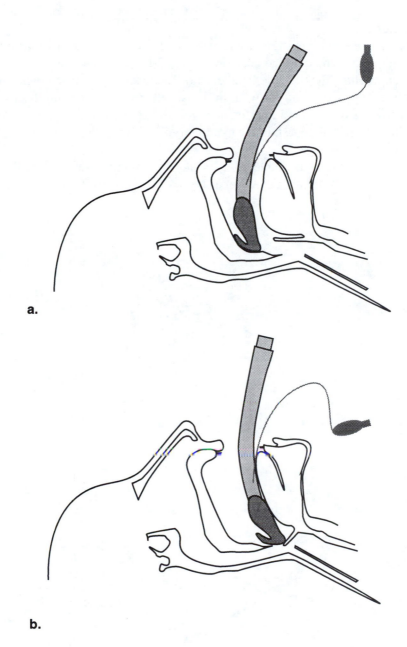

Fig. 13-4. When the LMA cushion curls (a) it impairs placement. It may push the epiglottis down over the larynx causing airway obstruction.

If there are no contraindications, tilt the patient's head into extension and slightly flex the neck.

Open the patient's mouth with your left hand and insert the LMA with your right (Fig. 13–5). The deflated cushion of the LMA should be directed posteriorly in the midline. Press the deflated cushion against the palate and then slide it down the posterior pharyngeal wall until resistence is felt. Pressing backwards and downwards helps avoid interference with the epiglottis. The LMA usually seats with the tip of the mask in the hypopharynx with the dark lines on the tube shaft opposite the front teeth.

Inflate the cushion (see Table 13-2) without holding the tube. The tube will typically move outward about 1-2 cm as the cuff centers itself around the laryn-

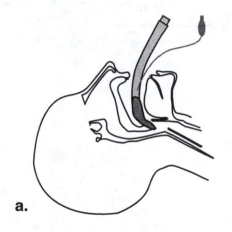

a.

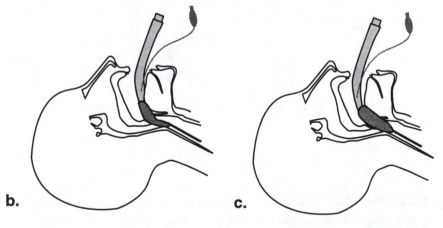

b.   **c.**

Fig. 13-5. Insertion of Laryngeal Mask Airway. Slide the LMA into the posterior pharynx until it seats against the larynx (a,b). Inflate cuff (c).

geal inlet. Watch the neck. You'll see the thyroid and cricoid cartilages rise. If it's hard to inflate the cushion, check the LMA's position (Fig. 13-6).

Inflating the cushion should provide a good seal around the larynx. It's common to have a leak at 15-20 cm H_2O with positive pressure ventilation. This often disappears with time as the soft tissue molds itself around the cushion. If

Table 11–2. Laryngeal Mask Cuff Inflation Volumes.	
Size 1:	2–5 cc
Size 2:	5–10 cc
Size 3:	10–25 cc
Size 4:	15–35 cc

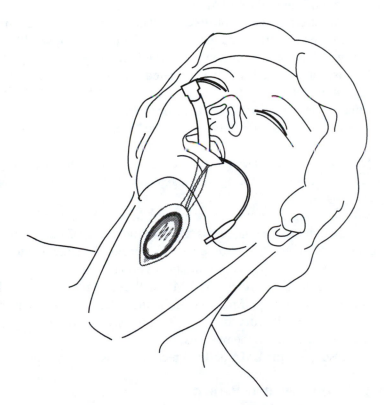

Fig. 13-6. The LMA in place

there is a leak at less than 15 cm H_2O then the LMA may be too small. Overinflation of the mask causes it to stiffen and lift away from the laryngeal inlet, often making the leak worse.

Make sure that the patient is ventilating adequately. If ventilation is inadequate try adding air to the cuff. If ventilation is still inadequate, then deflate the cuff and remove the tube. Ventilate the patient with bag and mask prior to another attempt.

The LMA does not protect against aspiration or regurgitation, although when properly seated no air should enter the stomach. The LMA does come in several sizes, including pediatric sizes, making it ideal for emergency failed intubations. It does not require an effective mask fit on the face or the maintence of good airway positioning. Thus it can be more easily used when the patient is being moved or is in an awkward position. It frees the provider's hands.

Problems With Positioning the LMA

Placement may be more difficult in patients with a large tongue or tonsils, a small mouth, or a "posterior" larynx since these anatomical features can cause malrotation or curling of the LMA.

Rotation of tube can lead to obstruction. The line on the tube should face upward and be in the midline of the upper lip of the patient. The LMA can be malpositioned with either downfolding or actual trapping of the epiglottis. This should be suspected if the LMA is not rotated but there is either obstruction or a poor seal with ventilation.

Although the technique described has been shown to be most frequently successful, occasionally an alternative technique to passing the LMA may work if the primary technique fails. Use your index finger to push the shaft or proximal connector into the hypopharynx. You can also place your index finger behind the lower part of the cushion to straighten the leading edge if it starts to curl (Fig. 13-7).

Partially inflating the cuff may help the LMA make the turn into the hypopharynx, although this technique has a higher incidence of folding the epiglottis down over the laryngeal inlet. Some providers insert the LMA upside down and then rotate it 180° while pushing it into the hypopharynx.

After many autoclave cycles, the LMA will get slightly softer and will lose its curvature. This can impair passage of the tube. A stylet can be used to stiffen the LMA and recreate its curvature. Don't let the stylet protrude beyond the grill of the mask or it can injure the pharynx.

You can also place the LMA under direct vision using laryngoscopy.

Caveats for the Pediatric Patient

There is less margin for error to correctly place an LMA in a neonate or small child. The larger tonsils of older children can interfere with insertion.

Difficulties in placement are more common. The LMA is more easily displaced, therefore correct placement and the ability to ventilate must be reverified whenever the child is moved.

Even when ideally positioned, gastric inflation and distention is possible if inflation pressure exceeds the cushion seal of about 20 cm H_2O.

Downfolding of the epiglottis is more common in children. Delayed airway obstruction has been reported in infants. Interference with ventilation is uncommon but it is recommended that you verify positioning with fiberoptic bronchoscopy, if possible, before using the LMA as a guide for intubation.

Cautions in the Use of the LMA

Because the LMA does not seal the trachea and because the esophageal opening may be present within the cushion 10–15% of the time, there is a risk of

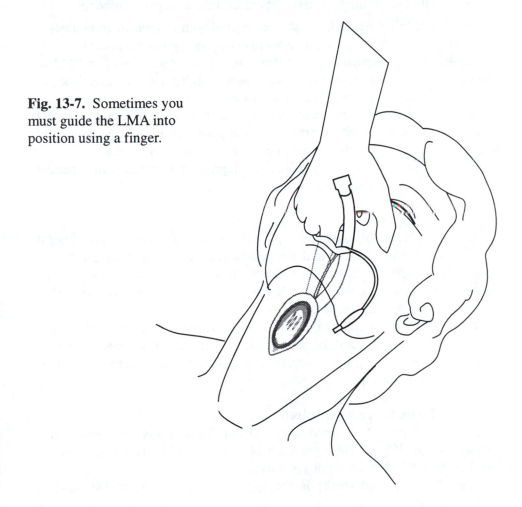

Fig. 13-7. Sometimes you must guide the LMA into position using a finger.

aspiration. The LMA is relatively contraindicated for use in:

- nonfasting patients
- morbid obesity
- pregnant patients over 14 weeks gestation
- acute abdomen
- hiatal hermia
- any abdominal condition with delayed gastric emptying
- acute trauma

There is risk of inadequate ventilation when used in patients with:

- thoracic injury
- massive or multiple injury
- poor pulmonary compliance (i.e. status asthmaticus, pneumothorax)

Therefore, at this time the LMA should be used with caution when intubation is not possible in the emergency, non-fasted patient or the trauma patient

Although better tolerated than an endotracheal tube, placement of an LMA in a conscious or semi-conscious patient can cause gagging and vomiting. The patient may also bite the provider during insertion.

Because ventilation is dependent on successfully sealing the hypopharyngeal space, the LMA is relatively contraindicated in patients with local pathology of the larynx and pharynx such as tumor, hematoma, abscess, or edema.

The LMA would not be very helpful in improving ventilation in a patient with obstruction below the glottis.

Removal of the LMA

The LMA is better tolerated by the patient than an endotracheal tube. Thus it is better to leave it in place until the patient regains full protective reflexes. Always suction the mouth well in order to clear any secretions on top of the cushion before removing the LMA. Deflate the cushion and remove the LMA. Avoid damaging the cushion on the teeth.

When used under anesthesia the LMA should be removed either with the patient completely anesthetized, or once awake. It should not be removed during Stage 2 of the awakening process when airway reflexes are heightened and laryngospasm may occur.

Use of the LMA to Assist Intubation

You can use the LMA as a guide for blind and fiberoptically directed endotracheal intubation. If good airway anesthesia is provided, the LMA can even be placed in the awake patient for this purpose.

If the LMA is placed ideally in the hypopharynx, the grill of the mask is directly over the laryngeal outlet and vocal cord aperture. Up to a size 6.0 cuffed endotracheal tube can be passed down the lumen of a size 3 or 4 LMA and into the trachea. A size 4.5 uncuffed tube can fit through a size 2 LMA. The ETT must be well lubricated. The endotracheal tube must be rotated 15–90° toward the left to allow the bevel to pass through the grill bars on the LMA. Once you feel the tube pass through the bars, at about 20 cm, then rotate it back and advance until the connector touches the LMA.

Cricoid pressure reduces the success rate. If you're holding cricoid pressure to protect against aspiration, consider transiently removing the pressure if you experience difficulty passing the tube.

The LMA can either be left in position around the endotracheal tube or it can be removed. This is sometimes difficult due to the tight fit between the tube and the inner wall of the LMA and due to the fact that there is no way to grip the tube as the LMA is backed out. One solution is to pass a fiberoptic scope down the tube into the trachea, thus allowing rapid re-intubation if the trachea is accidentally extubated. An intubating stylet or endotracheal tube changer can also be used blindly.

Another trick is to remove the endotracheal adaptor. Bundle the pilot balloon and its tubing over the top of the tube and into its shaft. Take the same size or one size smaller endotracheal tube and place its tip into the top of the tracheally placed tube. Use this to hold the tracheal tube steady as you slowly back the LMA out over it.

Whichever technique you choose, always re-verify continued tracheal placement of your endotracheal tube after LMA removal.

If the LMA is not located ideally, then the failure rate of blind intubation will increase. A fiberoptic bronchoscope can be used to visualize the larynx and thus ensure success. You can continously ventilate the patient during visualization (Fig. 13-8). Place the endotracheal tube into the LMA. Connect the tube to an angled connector with a rubber seal designed to allow fiberoptic bronchoscopy. Pass your well lubricated fiberoptic through the seal into the endotrachal tube to allow leisurely bronchoscopy. Once the trachea is intubated, you can remove the LMA before removing to fiberoptic cable to ensure that extubation does not occur.

A variation on this technqiue is to ventilate with the angled connector attached directly to the LMA. Pass the bronchoscope through the connector down the LMA into the trachea. A wire guide, such as a 0.0035 in Teflon coated, "floppy end" guide wire, such as a cardiac cath wire, can then be passed down the suction port of the fiberoptic into the trachea. The fiberoptic and LMA are removed over the wire and then the wire is used as a guide for the endotracheal tube. This technique would be especially useful for smaller endotracheal tubes such as pediatric tubes.

The emergency situation is a poor time to learn how to use the LMA to intubate. Practice on patients with normal airways when possible.

Care and Sterilization of the LMA

The LMA is designed for re-use. Since each LMA costs several hundred dollars, the only economical way to use LMAs at this time is to resterilize them between patients.

Soon after removal from the patient, the LMA should initally be washed with mild soap and water. Use a pipe cleaner style brush to clean secretions from the tube. Be careful not to damage the grill on the mask.

Then autoclave the LMA at a temperature no higher than 134°C for at least 3 minutes. **Never** use ethylene oxide, glutaraldehyde or formaldehyde. Make

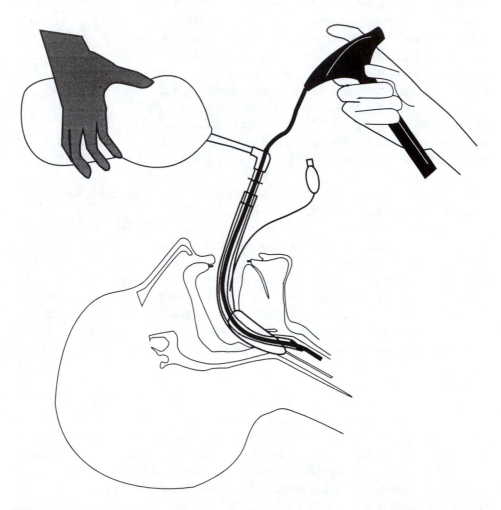

Fig. 13-8. Using the LMA as a guide for fiberoptic intubation. If the endotracheal tube is attached to an angled connector with a fiberoptic port, you can continue to ventilate during the intubation.

certain that the cushion and pilot tube are completely deflated before putting the LMA into the autoclave or they may burst from the heat induced expansion of air. If the drying cycle is omitted, between 100-250 re-uses have been possible, bringing the cost of the LMA per use into the same price range as an endotracheal tube.

Discard any LMA if it's discolored, damaged, or if you see abnormal bulging of the inflated cuff. Replacement valves are available if the valve leaks.

Esophageal-Tracheal Combitube

The Combitube (Sheridan Catheter Corp, Argyle, NY) is a double lumen ventilation tube for use during anesthesia and emergency airway management. The tube has 2 lumens, each with a 15mm airway connector at the proximal end (Fig. 13–9). There are 2 inflatable cuffs, a proximal 100cc latex pharyngeal cuff and a 15cc PVC cuff near the distal tip. Either lumen may be used to ventilate depending upon whether the tube lies in the esophagus or the trachea.

The Combitube is inserted either blindly or using direct laryngoscopy, entering the esophagus 98% of the time (Fig. 13–10). The proximal black rings should lie opposite the front teeth. Inflate the proximal balloon with 100 cc of air and the distal balloon with 15cc of air. Inflation of the proximal pharyngeal balloon normally causes the tube to move outward about 1 cm.

Next verify the location of the tube to determine which lumen should be used for ventilation. Since esophageal positioning is most likely, ventilate lumen 1 first. When positioned in the esophagus, air entering through the multiple side ports is trapped between the 2 cuffs and produces the positive pressure for chest inflation.

If ventilation is poor through lumen 1 then try lumen 2 since the Combitube may be in the trachea.

If ventilation continues to be poor then add more air to the proximal cuff since the seal may be inadequate. Try lumen 1 again. If the third attempt at ventilation fails remove the Combitube and ventilate the patient by bag and mask before trying this or another technique again.

There are several advantages of the Combitube over the EOA. Ventilation with the Combitube can occur regardless of whether the tube is in the esophagus or the trachea and the esophagus can be suctioned. Unlike the LMA, the Combitube provides some protection from aspiration.

A disadvantage of the Combitube is the lack of pediatric sizes.

Needle Cricothyroidotomy and Jet Ventilation

Needle cricothryoidotomy is a fast, easy way of providing oxygen to a patient with an obstructed airway who does not respond to more conventional means of opening the airway. It will buy you time to establish a more permanent airway such as an intubation or tracheostomy if the patient is hypoxic.

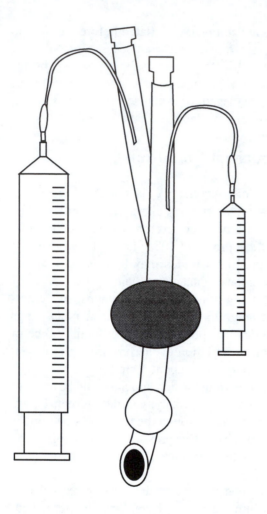

Fig. 13-9. Esophageal-Tracheal Combitude.

First identify the cricothyroid membrane by finding the cricoid ring. The membrane lies in the gap between the ring and the thyroid cartilage above it (Fig. 13–11). The membrane is about 10 mm high and 22 mm wide in the average adult. The vocal cords lie 1 cm above. The blood vessels tend to overlie the upper third of the cricothyroid membrane. Making your puncture in the lower third will minimize the risk of hitting them.

You can use any intravenous catheter-over-needle set to puncture the cricothyroid membrane. Use the largest catheter possible, such as a size 10 or 14 gauge in the adult. Attach a syringe to the hub of the needle and aspirate as you advance. Aim the needle slightly caudad. Your insertion should be slow and deliberate to avoid puncture of the posterior tracheal wall. The diameter of the adult trachea averages 18 mm. The aspiration of air verifies intra-tracheal placement.

Slide the catheter off the needle into the trachea. Again attach your syringe to

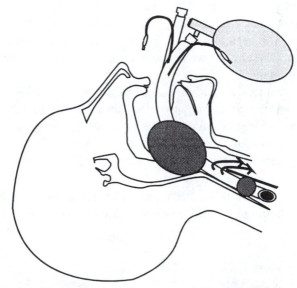

**COMBITUBE IN ESOPHAGUS. VENTILATE LUMEN #1.
AIR ENTERS TRACHEA FROM POSTERIOR PHARYNX.**

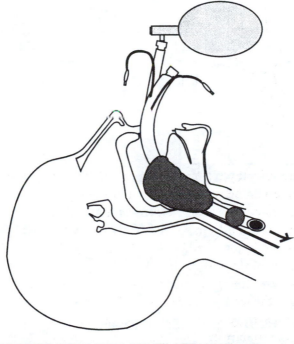

**COMBITUBE IN TRACHEA. VENTILATE LUMEN #2.
AIR ENTERS TRACHEA DIRECTLY.**

Fig. 13-10. Patterns of ventilation with the Esophageal-Tracheal Combitude.

the hub of the catheter and aspirate 10-20 cc of air to check placement and ensure free aspiration. It's essential that the catheter not be blocked by the tracheal wall or kinked. Jet ventilation against or into the tracheal wall can cause massive subcutaneous emphysema. Have an assistant steady the catheter by the hub to ensure that it doesn't move.

You now need to connect the catheter to a ventilation system. Because of the small diameter, the best means of giving oxygen through this device is a jet ventilator with a Sander's valve. When using the jet it is imperative that the airway be at least partially open above the cricothyroid membrane. If not, the gas pressure will build and potentially cause a pneumothorax. Misplacement of the catheter can lead to subcutaneous emphysema.

If a jet ventilator is unavailable, then there are several ways to connect the catheter to your ventilation system. The connector from a number 3 endotracheal

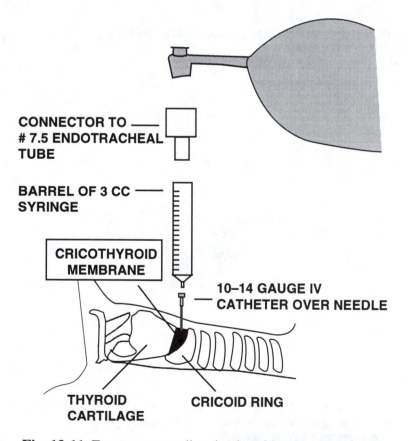

CONNECTOR TO
 # 7.5 ENDOTRACHEAL
TUBE

BARREL OF 3 CC
SYRINGE

CRICOTHYROID
MEMBRANE

10–14 GAUGE IV
CATHETER OVER NEEDLE

THYROID
CARTILAGE

CRICOID RING

Fig. 13-11. Emergency needle cricothyroidotomy and a means of connecting it to a ventilation system.

tube fits snugly into the hub of any intravenous catheter. However, this tiny assemply is often difficult to hold while squeezing the bag. I prefer to place the connector from a number 7.5 endotracheal tube into the barrel of a 3 cc syringe. The barrel of the syringe now mates to the hub of your catheter and gives you something more substantial to hold. You can also place an endotracheal tube within the barrel of a ten cc syringe and inflates the cuff to maintain the connection. You must ventilate vigorously to pass enough oxygen through the catheter. Gas will escape through the mouth.

Another technique is to attach the barrel from a tuberculin syringe to the catheter hub and connect this to oxygen tubing. If the oxygen tubing can then be connected to the fresh gas outflow from an anesthesia machine a "jet" can be jury rigged.

Reports indicate that patients can maintain themselves for several minutes breathing spontaneously through a 10g catheter. Although hypoxia is avoided hypercarbia will develop. However, any oxygen supplied during emergency treatment of airway obstruction is useful.

Surgical Cricothyroidotomy

Surgical cricothyroidotomy is more hazardous than needle cricothyroidotomy. Unlike jet venilation, it can be used when total upper airway obstruction is present. It allows for insertion of a larger tube, thus improving ease of ventilation. Suctioning of the airway is possible. Finally, it can be secured and left in place for a longer period, while the transtracheal catheter must be replaced relatively quickly with a more definitive airway.

The indictions for surgical cricothyoidotomy are:

- "can't ventilate/can't intubate" scenario;
- upper airway foreign body or other obstruction;
- severe trauma to face and mouth;
- traumatic C-spine injury where oral intubation not feasible.

Consult an experienced surgeon to perform or to assist you with this procedure unless a delay will jeopardize patient survival.

Find the cricoid membrane and prep the skin. Use local anesthesia if you have time. Pull the skin tight and make a shallow incision over the cricoid membrane. Dissect bluntly and rapidly down to the membrane (Fig. 13-12a). Take care to avoid the large superficial veins and the thyroid gland. Crico–thyroidotomy is fairly bloodless if you don't damage these vessels.

Make a stab wound about 1-1.5 cm long in the cricoid membrane with a number 11 blade. Twist the blade to allow ventilation (Fig. 13-12b).

Pull the cricoid ring upward with a tracheal hook or a clamp. This opens the trachea and allows insertion of a tracheostomy or endotracheal tube (Fig. 13-12c). If the incision is too small, use curved scissors or a tracheal dilator to

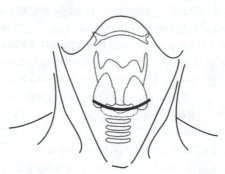

a. MAKE TRANSVERSE INCISION THROUGH SKIN. DISSECT RAPIDLY DOWN TO CRICOID MEMBRANE.

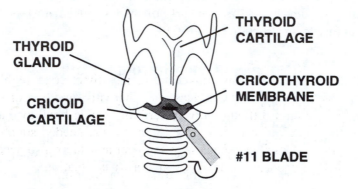

b. MAKE STAB WOUND IN CRICOID MEMBRANE WITH #11 BLADE. TWIST BLADE TO ENLARGE HOLE.

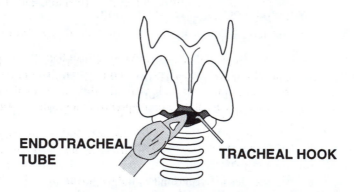

c. PULL CRICOID RING FORWARD WITH HOOK OR CLAMP. INSERT ENDOTRACHEAL TUBE.

Fig. 13-12. Surgical cricothyroidotomy.

bluntly spread the opening. Check breath sounds immediately to make sure your tube lies in the trachea and not the subcutaneous tissue.

Potential complications from this emergency procedure include injury to the larynx, hemorrhage into the trachea, aspiration, pneumothorax, esophageal damage, and subcutaneous or mediastinal emphysema. *Death* from asphyxia — from failure or from improper placement of the tube — can also occur. Use surgical cricothyroidotomy with great care.

Several kits are now marketed for non-surgeon providers to allow easy and quick placement of a surgical cricothyroidotomy. NU-TRACH™ (Bivone Medical Technologies; Gary, Ind.), Melker Emergency Crico–thyrotomy Catheter Set™ (Cook Critical Care), and the Arndt Emergency Cricothyrotomy Catheter Set™ (Cook Critical Care) are three such devices. These kits contain all of the instruments needed to provide an emergency airway.

Due to the greater complexity of the surgery and the increased risk of complications tracheostomy is beyond the scope of this book.

Emergency Airway Cart

Emergency airway situations can occur at any time. It is highly recommended that each provider know at least one alternative method of securing a failed airway. Having a difficult "airway cart" or "tackle box" available saves precious minutes in an airway emergency since all the needed supplies are together and readily accessible. Needless to say your assistants also need to know where it's stored so they can fetch it for you in a crisis situation.

Further Reading

Benumof JL, Scheller MS. The importance of transtracheal jet ventilation in the management of the difficult airway. *Anesth.* 1989; 71: 769–778.

Benumof JL: Use of the laryngeal mask airway to facilitate fibersope-aided tracheal intubation. *Anesth Analg* 1992;74: 313–315.

Biebuyck JF: The Laryngeal Mask Airway, its uses in anesthesiology. *Anesth.* 1993; 79: 144-163.

Brimacombe J, Berry A: Insertion of the Laryngeal Mask Airway — A Prospective Study of four Techniques" *Anaesth Intensi Care* 1993; 21: No. 1: 89– 92.

Hankins DG, Carruthers N, Frascone RJ, et al: Complication rates for the esophageal obturator airway and the endotracheal tube in the prehospital setting. *Prehospital and Disaster Medicine* 1993; 8:117–120.

Heard MB, Caldicott LD, Fletcher JE, Selsby DS: Fiberoptic guided endotracheal intubation via the Laryngeal Mask Airway in pediatric patients: a report of a series. *Anesth Analg* 1996; 82:1287-9

McEwan AI, Mason DG: The laryngeal mask airway. *J Clin. Anesth.* 1993; 4: 252–257.

Pennant JH, Walker MB: Comparison of the endotracheal tube and laryngeal mask in airway management by paramedical personnel. *Anesth Analg* 1992; 74:531–534.

Wissler RN: The esophageal-tracheal combitube. *Anesthesiology Review* 1993; XX No. 4: 147–152.

14 SPECIALIZED INTUBATING EQUIPMENT

In previous chapters, we discussed intubation using the standard equipment readily available in operating rooms, emergency rooms, ambulances, and cardiac arrest carts. Anesthesiologists, intensive care specialists, and surgeons occasionally use more specialized equipment to intubate patients with difficult airways.

Safeguarding Patient Safety

Since it's easy to loose track of time when performing any of the following maneuvers, use the following safety precautions.

Monitor the patient's oxygenation. Observe the patient's color. If you have a pulse oximeter, use it to measure the patient's oxygen saturation. Keep the O_2 saturation above 90%, corresponding to a PO_2 above 60 mmHg. You'll need arterial blood gases to tell you the exact PO_2 and PCO_2 and thus identify hypoventilation, hypercarbia, and hypoxemia. However, even in a large hospital these results often take more than 10-15 minutes to arrive — sometimes too late to help in a crisis. Always provide extra oxygen when available.

Have your assistant time any period of apnea occurring during airway instrumentation. If it takes more than one or two minutes to perform any maneuver in the apneic patient, stop and ventilate. Let any awake patient "catch his breath" during a prolonged attempt. It helps him or her tolerate the procedure better and gives you a chance to gather your thoughts. Have an assistant monitor vital signs while you concentrate on the airway. High blood pressure and fast heart rates harm some patients as much as the lack of oxygen .

Tell the patient what you're doing. Be supportive. Cooperative patients make intubation safer and easier.

Suction the airway frequently. Gagging on the instruments can cause vomiting and even an alert patient can aspirate. After intubation, suction the endotracheal tube well.

Use sedation and local anesthesia judiciously, but watch for complications and overdose (see Chapter 15).

Discuss problems with more experienced intubators and ask for their advice and help. Asking for help during intubation should never threaten your ego. Asking for assistance only helps your patient.

It is highly recommended that you practice any of these specialized techniques on healthy patients with normal airways before trying them in an emergency.

Flexible Guides

Endotracheal tubes often enter the esophagus during difficult intubations because they don't curve enough to enter an anterior larynx. You can sometimes enter the larynx with an LTA (laryngotracheal anesthesia kit), and then use it as a guide for threading the endotracheal tube. An LTA is simply a lidocaine-filled syringe attached to a long, stiff, curved catheter. It's normally used to squirt lidocaine down the trachea to prevent wheezing or hypertension during intubation. Place the LTA beside the endotracheal tube and insert it through the Murphy eye *from the outside* (Fig. 14-1). Aim the catheter upward into the larynx and then slide the endotracheal tube over it and into the trachea. You can substitute a stylet for the LTA. Be very gentle in order to avoid damaging the trachea.

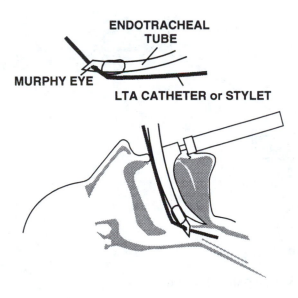

ENDOTRACHEAL TUBE

MURPHY EYE

LTA CATHETER or STYLET

Fig. 14-1. LTA or Stylet through the Murphy eye.

An endotracheal tube exchanger (Fig. 14-2) is a long, flexible tube similar in size to a nasogastric tube. It's used to exchange endotracheal tubes by sliding down the lumen of the old tube and acting as a stent for the new one. It can also be used to assist intubation. When the endotracheal tube won't pass into the trachea, you can thread the tube exchanger down the lumen and into the trachea. Then use the exchanger as a stent to complete the insertion of the endotracheal tube.

The Flexguide NCC (Fig. 14-3) consists of a barrel with a thumb ring plunger, attached to a long, thin rod about 6 cm (2.5 inches) longer than an endotracheal

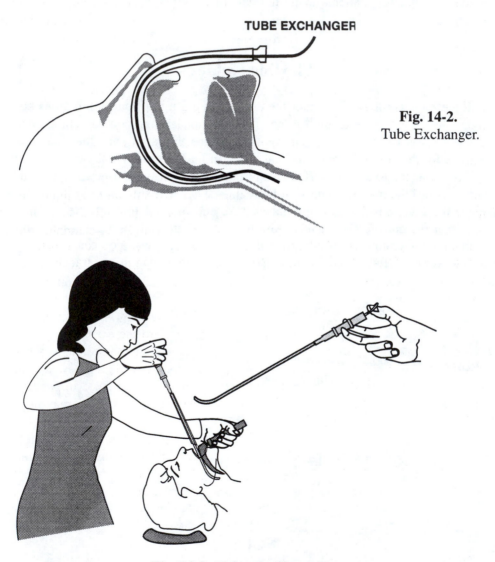

TUBE EXCHANGER

Fig. 14-2.
Tube Exchanger.

Fig. 14-3. Using the Flexguide.

tube. Pushing the plunger curves the tip of the rod up. Insert the rod into your tube until the barrel seats into the 15 mm adapter, allowing them to act as a unit. Perform routine direct laryngoscopy and aim the tip of the rod into the larynx, maneuvering the tip as necessary. The Flexguide is often awkward to use because the right hand is at operator eye level. Keep your arm and back straight to minimize this problem. Standing on a stool helps.

Whenever you intubate without seeing the vocal cords, immediately check proper tube placement. Esophageal intubation easily occurs.

A fiberoptic intubating stylet now exists which allows direct visualization through an eyepiece of the view at the tip of the stylet. The larynx can be directly seen and entered and the stylet used as a guide for tube placement. The stylet is as malleable as a standard stylet and may be curved into the usual shapes used in routine intubation. It should not be bent into sharp angles which would damage the fiberoptic bundles.

The gum-elastic bougie is an endotracheal introducer which is made of a braided polyester base with a resin coating, giving it both flexibility and stiffness at body temperature. The standard size for intubation is 15Fr, which is 60 cm long. It will retain the curvature given to it, making it very useful for anterior airways.

The gum-elastic bougie is stiff enough to cause damage or perforation of the trachea and bronchi and must be used with caution. It should be used in combination with laryngoscopy under direct vision rather than as a blind stent. It is not recommended for use for exchanging endotracheal tubes. A standard tube exchanger should be used for this purpose since the lumen is hollow and will allow insufflation or jetting of oxygen if necessary. The technique described below can be performed using an endotracheal tube exchanger, although this device won't hold a specific curve or shape.

Following laryngoscopy, the bougie is passed forward toward the probable location of the laryngeal opening. Correct placement into the trachea is felt as "clicks" as the bougie slides over tracheal rings. The bougie may rotate as it encounters the main stem bronchus or stop when the smaller bronchi are reached. It should not be forced. The bougie and laryngoscope are then fixed in position and the endotracheal tube is passed down over the bougie. The tube may need to be rotated to allow passage through the vocal cords. You then withdraw the bougie and laryngoscope and verify correct placement of the tube.

A recent study (Nolan) in patients requiring cervical spine precautions and stabilization showed that in the neutral position, the view of the larynx on direct laryngoscopy was reduced in 45% of the patients. Of these, 22% had views showing only the epiglottis. The patients in the bougie group were all successfully intubated within 15-20 seconds. On the other hand 5 patients in the laryngoscopy only group subsequently required the bougie and 5 required more than 50 seconds for intubation. Thus the bougie appears to be a good adjunct for difficult intubations. You should practice its use in normal patients to gain experience before you need it in an emergency. An epiglottis only view can be simulated by laryngoscope placement.

Light wands or stylets work by trans-illuminating the trachea at the point of the sternal notch. With the trachea thus identified, the stylet is then used as a guide for the endotracheal tube. Typical lighted stylets are self contained, with a small power source the size of a pen flashlight attached to a long, thin, somewhat stiff stylet. Lighted stylets are designed for re-use.

To use, make sure the light source is functional. Lubricate the stylet well to allow it slide easily. Then place the stylet into the endotracheal tube. Make sure that the tip does not extend past the tip or through the Murphy eye or tissue trauma can occur. Like any stylet/tube combination, bend the tip 90° into a "hockey stick" shape.

Uncover the anterior neck and place the bed at a height where it can easily be seen. You might consider dimming the room lights to improve visibility. Turn on the light and insert the tube/stylet unit into the mouth. As the tip of the stylet approaches the larynx you will begin to see the light through the skin of the anterior neck. Cricoid pressure may help. When the stylet enters the trachea, a bright, discrete light will continue down the *midline* in a straight line toward the sternal notch where it disappears. Thread the endotracheal tube and remove the stylet.

When the stylet enters the esophagus the light will not be seen or will be very hazy and dim. When the stylet enters the pyriform sinuses you will see a widespread, diffuse glow on either side of the midline. The goal is to keep the light midline. Any blind technique can theoretically cause tissue trauma. Be gentle.

Lighted stylets have several disadvantages including:

* require a blind approach;
* difficult in patients with anterior or traumatized airways;
* difficult in obese patients;
* can't be used in children needing an ETT < 5.

Manipulating Endotracheal
Tubes, Blades and Handles

Nasal endotracheal tubes sometimes enter the esophagus because they won't curve forward enough after entering the oropharynx. Several devices and techniques help solve this problem.

Endotrol tubes have a pull cord attached to a ring near the 15 mm adapter. Pulling the ring turns the tip of the tube anteriorly, allowing you to manipulate the tip with more precise control.

Having an assistant use a **hook** to pull the tip of the tube forward during nasal intubation also works (Fig. 14-4.)

Tube benders grab the tube *behind the cuff* and bend it upward when you close the jaws.

Many variations on laryngoscope blades and handles exist. The **polio blade** (Fig. 14-5) was invented to intubate polio patients inside an "iron lung." Encasing the patient's body in a machine made conventional laryngoscopy difficult — you couldn't extend the head or position the handle over the chest. The polio blade is a straight blade which attaches to the handle at an angle of nearly 180°. Positioning the handle over the patient's head changes the angle of lift. You usually don't need to tilt the head to see the larynx — useful in neck-injured patients. Don't lever the blade against the upper teeth, lift the mandible away from you.

A **Howland lock** (Fig. 14-6) fits onto the top of the standard handle. It

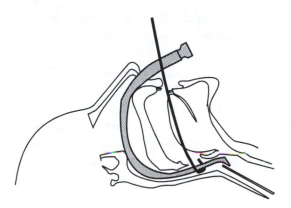

Fig. 14-4. Using a hook to help pass a tube with too little curvature.

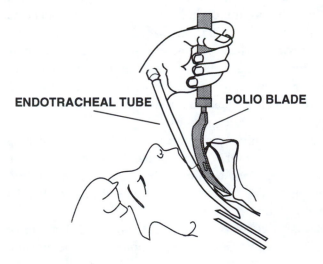

ENDOTRACHEAL TUBE   POLIO BLADE

Fig. 14-5. Using the polio blade. Don't press on the teeth.

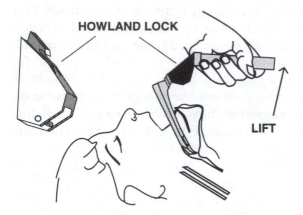

HOWLAND LOCK

LIFT

Fig. 14-6. The Howland Lock increases the angulation of the blade and improves mechanical advantage.

increases the angle of the blade, allowing you to lift the blade more forcefully without levering on the teeth. The angulation of the lock makes it more awkward to use in a barrel-chested patient.

Some handles let you vary the angle of the blade from a sharp bend to complete extension, based on the clinical situation.

Huffman Prisms attach to the MacIntosh blade, bending the image so you see about 30° farther into the larynx. The image is right-side up. Knowing the exact location of the larynx helps aim the endotracheal tube (Fig. 14-7). The prism will fog if not warmed beforehand — easily done by immersion in hot water or storage in your pocket.

The Augustine Guide (Augustine Medical) is a 2 piece device. The first piece consists of a special plastic positioning blade connected to a handle with a channel guide to hold an endotracheal tube. The second piece, or Augustine Stylet, has a "S" shaped molded tip with 6 aspiration holes, 3 on each side, connected to a 35cc syringe esophageal detection system (Fig. 14-8).

The kit is designed for use with the head in a neutral position and thus may be useful in the patient needing cervical spine precautions. Like the laryngoscope it may be used in the conscious or unconscious patient, although the conscious patient should optimally receive topical anesthesia to prevent gagging. It can be used in patients trapped in awkward positions.

Before inserting the Augustine Guide, place the well lubricated intubating stylet through a size 7-8.0 endotracheal tube. Advance the "S" shaped tip to the edge of the endotracheal tube opening and then insert both the tube and the stylet into the channel of the Guide. The tip of the endotracheal tube and stylet should be under the positioning blade.

Advance the tongue anteriorly, either by grabbing it with a 4X4 gauze or with a tongue blade. Slide the Augustine Guide into position so that the indentation in its leading edge straddles the hyoepiglottic ligament, which extends from the epiglottis to the hyoid bone. This places its tip in the vallecula. The handle is 90° to the plane of the face. If in proper position, moving the Guide from side to side will cause the hyoid bone to move, a movement which can be felt through the neck tissue (Fig. 14-9).

Now advance the stylet and syringe as a unit until the syringe meets the endotracheal tube connector. The stylet should move easily without obstruction. If in the trachea, you will be able to aspirate 30-35 cc's of air with no problem.

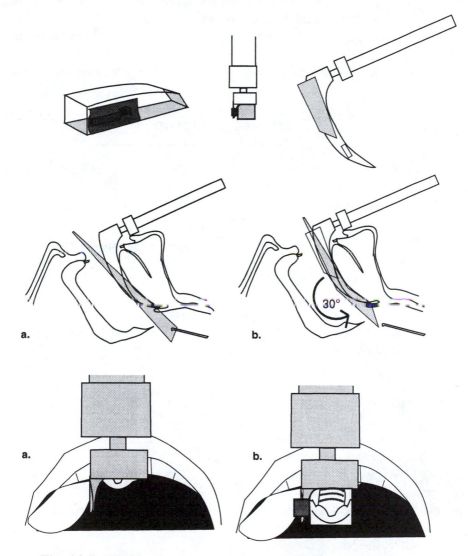

Fig. 14-7. The Huffman Prism brings an anterior larynx into view.

When you release the plunger there should be no recoil. The presence of resistance to aspiration or of recoil of the plunger indicate probable esophageal placement and stylet should be withdrawn to try again.

Once the stylet is in the trachea, hold the handle firmly and release the tube and stylet from the channel. Advance the tube over the stylet into the trachea. You may need to rotate the endotracheal tube around the stylet to get the tube to pass through the vocal cords.

Use caution in the patient who has a distended stomach for any reason since this may allow you to aspirate air through the stylet. This could fool you into thinking that an esophageal intubation was in the trachea.

The Augustine Guide can be used without the stylet for blind intubation and to also assist fiberoptic intubation.

With any of these techniques, always verify correct endotracheal tube place-

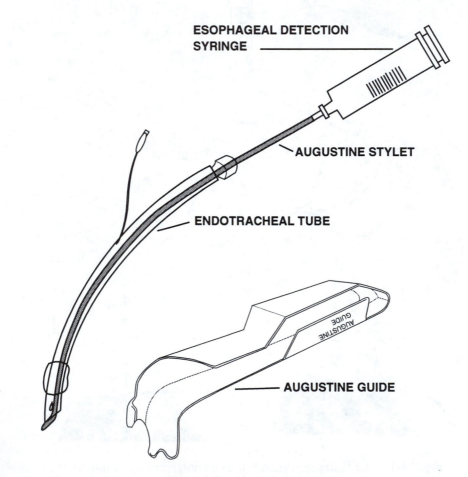

Fig. 14-8. Augustine Guide.

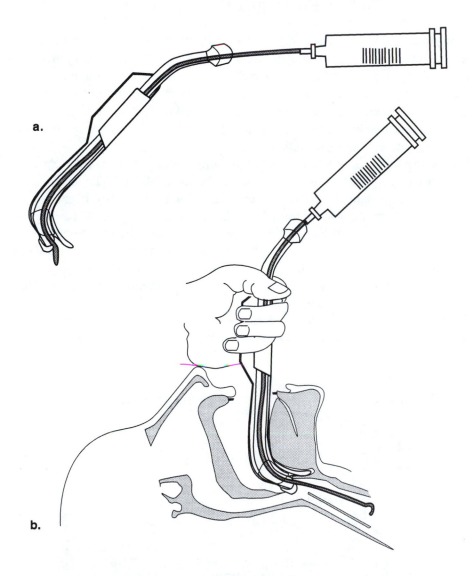

Fig. 14-9. Augustine Guide and Stylet. a: Endotracheal tube and Augustine Stylet positioned in channel of Augustine Guide; b: Esophageal Detection Syringe used to identify the trachea. Air is freely aspirated with no syringe plunger recoil. Note type og guide in vallecula. Note tip of guide in vallecula.

ment by listening for breath sounds over chest and stomach and by identifying the presence of CO_2 if possible. Esophageal intubation can easily occur during blind placement in the patient with a difficult airway

Flexible Fiberoptic Bronchoscopes

Many anesthesia services and intensive care units use fiberoptic broncho-scopes regularly for difficult intubations. Bronchoscopy is harder than direct la-ryngoscopy because bronchoscopes have several controls for manipulating the angle of the tip; because the narrow angle of view makes interpretation of the image more difficult; and because they are awkward to hold while maneuvering the tube. These instruments often cost in excess of $1000 and are easily dam-aged if you ignore certain precautions.

The device consists of a long cable containing bundles of threadlike glass fi-bers connected to a pistol grip handle holding the control knobs. The handle atta-ches to a portable light source by another long cable (Fig. 14-10). Light travels down the glass bundles with minimal loss in brightness because of the internal reflection within the glass threads. The image returns along the same route.

Since the fiberoptic bundles are glass, *never* bend the cables or wrap them tightly around your hand. Holding the cable in a single *loose* coil avoids break-age. Don't pile equipment on top of the scope. Train anyone who has to clean the scope how to avoid breakage.

First, attach the light source. Look through the viewfinder and focus the lens by aiming the tip at some printed text. Note the distance of the object from the tip of the cable when the image focuses. Hold the lens cable straight and gently

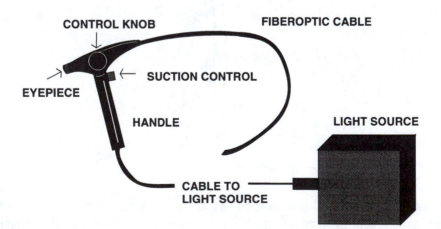

Fig. 14-10. The fiberoptic bronchoscope.

turn the control knob. Memorize which way the cable curves when you turn the knob (Fig. 14-11). Most viewfinders will have an assymetric mark on the perimeter of the image field. This mark allows you to remain oriented to the direction of the tip movement in relationship to the larynx. Remind yourself before each use of the orientation of this mark to the intended movement of the tip.

The unprepared lens will fog. Apply an antifogging solution. A dab of mineral oil or antifogging soap works well. Use hibiclens if antifogging soap is not available. Don't use solvents which can dissolve the glue holding the bundles together. Dry the lens tip carefully to avoid scratching it.

Preparation of the patient is important — if time permits. Sedation, topicalization, and the administration of a drying agent such as glycopyrrolate (Robinul) or atropine will provide you with a more cooperative patient and a superior working situation. Use a nasal vasocontrictor with nasal intubations to reduce the risk of nose bleeds (see Chapter 10). As these medications will take several minutes to work give them ahead of time if possible. Recommendations for the safe use of sedatives and local anesthestics are described elsewhere in the text.

Choose the largest tube you can as this eases cable insertion and avoids damage. Too small a tube may wrinkle the cable's plastic covering. On the other hand, a pediatric cable may not be stiff enough to guide a large tube. An adult scope will fit any tube 6.5 mm (26 Fr.) or larger. A pediatric scope will fit inside a 4.5 mm (20 Fr.) or larger tube. Lubricate the cable with K-Y jelly or lidocaine ointment by spreading lubricant with a gauze pad from a point about 5 cm (2 inches) from the tip back toward the handle. Lubricant on the lens will blur the image.

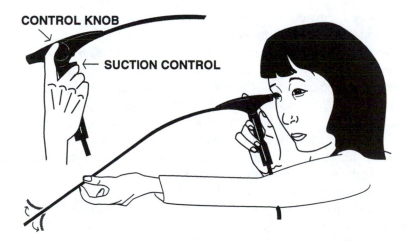

Fig. 14-11. Practice with the controls *before* inserting the bronchoscope.

Fiberoptic bronchoscopy allows intubation of both conscious and unconscious patients. Awake intubation lets patients breathe and protect their own airway.

The availability of two suction aparatuses is helpful. The first allows direct suctioining of the airway as needed. The second should be attached to the suction port of the bronchoscope. The end of the suction tubing must frequently be cut to allow connection to this port so prepare it ahead of time. Suction the airway frequently during the intubation. Instrumentation of the oropharynx, sedation, and local anesthesia of the airway predispose to aspiration — *even when your patient is awake.*

You can either stand at the head of the bed, in the usual intubating position, or at the side of the patient, facing back toward the head. There are advantages and disavantages to each. (Fig. 14-12a). Standing at the head gives the operator the anatomical relations in the standard intubating position. Left and right, up and down are unchanged. The disadvantage of this postion is that the multiple angles that the bronchoscope is forced to make in its journey through the oropharynx hamper the maneuverability of the tip.

When you stand at the patient's side facing the head (Fig. 14-12b), the directions for controlling the tip are reversed. From the side, aiming toward the patient's left means turning the cable tip to *your* right. Aiming anteriorly means turning the tip down instead of up. In this instance using the assymetric marker visible in the viewfinder to keep you oriented to direction becomes very helpful. Once the directional changes are mastered, it's often easier to perform fiberoptic bronchscopy from this side position because the cable doesn't have to make as many turns. It's therefore easier to manipulate the tip.

Because of the flexibility of the cable, rigid guides are often used to help direct its movement. For example, several types of oral airways, the Ovassapian and the Airway Intubator, are often used. These airways have a large channel down the center which hold the endotracheal tube and the enclosed fiberoptic cable fairly steady so that the tip can be manipulated. These airways also protect your expensive cable from the patient's teeth. During nasotracheal intubation the nasotracheal tube can act as the guide. Never be afraid to turn or reposition the guide to allow better placement of the cable to enhance your aim. The guide should play an active role in the intubation. Proper placement can make intubation easy. Misplacement of the guide can completely prevent intubation.

Insert the cable into the endotracheal tube. If the tube is small, removing the endotracheal tube adaptor may improve the fit.

For oral intubations the tube may be slid up the cable out or your way or placed within the mouth or airway guide. Use of the endotracheal tube as part of your guide can improve control.

For nasal intubations the tube may either be advanced through the nose until it just turns into the posterior pharynx or kept back on the cable. There are advantages and disadvantages to both. Keeping it out of the nose until the trachea is cannulated may sometimes improve maneuverability of the cable, but it risks being subsequently unable to pass the tube through the nose if the tube is too large. First placing the tube through the nose can be helpful, because it allows the tube to act as your guide and it verifies that the tube will fit. On the other hand, you risk nose bleed, which can profoundly interfere with your ability to use the fiberoptic.

Hold the cable in the left hand and the pistol grip control in the right, using either your right thumb or index finger to turn the control knob. Keep the cable fairly taught and straight. Hold it with both hands to let it to turn as a unit. The cable is very flexible. If allowed to loop you'll lose control of the tip and be unable to direct its placement. You should also plan to rotate the scope head with your arm and shoulder, not just your hand, to change direction. This permits must greater range of motion and control of the tip. Don't expect to find the larynx by just flexing the tip.

Dimming the room lights slightly may improve your image — if lower lighting doesn't compromise patient safety. A short intubator may prefer to stand on a step-stool.

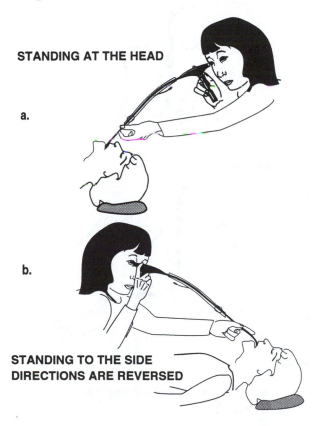

STANDING AT THE HEAD

a.

b.

STANDING TO THE SIDE
DIRECTIONS ARE REVERSED

Fig. 14-12. Keep back and arm straight for bronchoscopy positioning.

Put the cable into the patient's mouth. Have the patient stick his or her tongue out or have your assistant gently pull the patient's tongue forward if the tongue is in the way. Advance the cable while looking into the eyepiece. Identify structures as you see them (Fig. 14-13). Make certain the tip isn't in the tube when you flex it or the threads may break. Also watch to make sure the cable exits the tube *tip*, not the Murphy eye. If necessary, to improve your aim rotate or reposition the distal end of the endotracheal tube or move your guide. Pass the lens through the vocal cords when you see them. However, return the tip to neutral position before you advance it down the trachea. The image blurs during the passage through the vocal cords. A clear image of the tracheal rings appears on the other side and you'll see the carina if you advance far enough. Hold the instrument steady and slide the tube down the cable using it as a guide. If the tube won't pass, rotate it gently to allow the tip to slide off the anterior commissure. Remove the cable, attach your 15 mm adapter and oxygen source, and ventilate. Check breath sounds.

When you can't identify landmarks withdraw slightly to look at the big

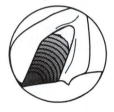 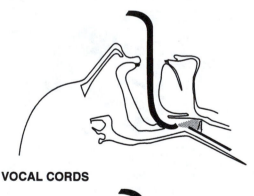

VOCAL CORDS

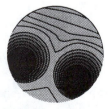 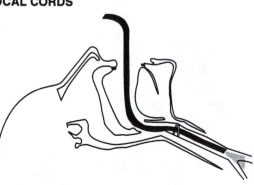

CARINA

Fig. 14-13. Practice with the controls *before* inserting the bronchoscope.

picture. Make sure your cable is actually headed toward the oropharynx. Sometimes it can be twisted around and misdirected into the nasopharynx, giving a confusing picture of the turbinates and choanae. Reposition the head as needed, maintaining cervcial precautions if appropriate.

Oral fiberoptic intubation in edentulous patients can occasionally be hard. Without the teeth to stabilize it, the oral guide tends to position itself against the back of the pharynx. This not only can block the advancement of the fiberoptic or tube but also changes the angle of approach to glottic opening. Pushing the endotracheal tube into the mouth tends to shove both guide and tube back against the wall of the pharynx. Have your assistant hold the oral guide forward in a more standard position. You may find it helpful in this situation to keep the tube back on the cable, and first advancing only the cable into the guide and trachea.

If the cable won't pass into the trachea despite a clear field of view it's often because the angle it must turn is too sharp. Pull back the endotracheal tube or otherwise reposition the guides or the patient's head and try again. Try switching to the other nostril. Change from the oral to the nasal approach or vice versa. Keep your options open.

When an intubating oral airway is not available you can use anything leading to the base of the tongue to guide you to the larynx. For example, a MacIntosh blade held by your assistant holds the anatomy in good position. Simply follow the curve with the tip of the cable.

With dimmed room lights, you'll actually see the light shining through the neck as the tip nears the larynx. As the cable enters the trachea the light moves down toward the chest and disappears. Failure to see the light as the cable advances may mean esophageal placement.

Inability to identify landmarks may mean the scope lies in the esophagus. Pull the cable back until recognizable landmarks appear. You'll see a grey tunnel when the lens is inside the tube.

Always use gentle technique. It's often better to start with the fiberoptic bronchoscope whenever you think you might eventually need to use it. Multiple prior attempts at blind intubation may bloody the airway and make identification of structures difficult.

You can ventilate with a nasal airway plus endotracheal tube adapter (Fig.14-14). An assistant ventilates while sealing the mouth and nares around the instrument. This technique can be used on apneic patients and also to maintain deep anesthesia during intubation under general anesthesia. Always have someone verify ventilation by listening to breath sounds. Don't rely on chest movement alone. After intubation, suction the endotracheal tube to remove secretions or blood.

An LMA can also be used to ventilate while acting as a guide for intubation while using the fiberoptic. This technique is described in Chapter 13.

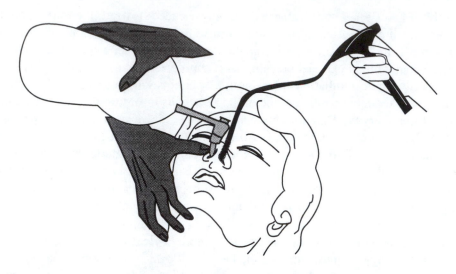

Fig. 14-14. Ventilation with a nasal airway and Ambu bag.

Use of the fiberoptic bronchoscope requires practice and emergencies are a poor time to learn the skill. If you have a fiberoptic, practice intubating the mannikin. You can apply clay or other obstructions in the airway to mimic the difficult intubation. Anesthesia and surgical personnel can use it during routine intubation of patients with normal airways scheduled for elective surgery. Don't wait until you need it to use it.

Retrograde Wires

A wire or catheter — passed through the cricothyroid membrane and advanced up into the oropharynx — can act as a guide for the endotracheal tube. You may perform the procedure with the patient awake or asleep. Only use this method if you can ventilate the patient during the intubation, because it takes several minutes to perform. When you can't ventilate, an emergency cricothyroidotomy or tracheostomy makes more sense. Contraindications include coagulation abnormalities, extensive subglottic tumor growth, inability to identify the cricoid membrane due to tumor, skin infiltration, or scar tissue.

Identify the cricothyroid membrane and clean the skin with antiseptic. If time and patient condition permit use transtracheal lidocaine (see Chapter 15) after a skin wheal of lidocaine with epinephrine to reduce skin bleeding. The guide catheter must be long enough to pass up the trachea, out the oropharynx, and then through the entire length of an endotracheal tube. A 0.035 cm ga. 145 cm vascular guide wire works well when passed through an 18-14g IV catheter.

Other choices include a self-contained long-line CVP kit, or an epidural needle and catheter. Any wire should have a soft, flexible tip if possible.

Attach your IV cather or needle to a syringe and aim the bevel toward the patient's head. Aspirate air as you enter the trachea through the cricothyroid membrane and then hold the needle firmly. Detach the syringe and thread the wire through the IV catheter (Fig. 14-15). The wire will usually pass out the mouth or nose although it can go down to the carina or coil in the posterior pharynx. Use Magill forceps to pull the wire when you see it. Have an assistant firmly hold the end of the wire. Be gentle to avoid trauma or pneumothorax.

For oral intubations, pass the wire through the Murphy eye from *outside* in. Push it up the tube until it exits at the top. Hold the wire tense. Slide your endotracheal tube down the wire. The tip should enter the larynx and stop when the Murphy eye is level with the catheter's entrance hole and the tip is about 2 cm below the vocal cords. Hold the tube securely, pull the wire out of the tube from below, and advance the tube down the trachea. Check proper placement.

Sometimes the guidewire will pass out the nose on its own. If it doesn't — and you desire a nasal intubation — pull the guidewire through the mouth as described. Pass a cut NG tube or large bore suction catheter through the nose into the posterior pharynx and out the mouth. Pass the wire up through it and out the nose. Insert the guide catheter into the lumen of the endotracheal tube and advance the tube into the trachea. In this situation, the tip of the endotracheal tube will lie level with the catheter's entrance hole, about 1 cm below the cords. Hold the tube securely, withdraw the wire, and advance the tube. Again, check proper placement.

You can make the guidewire stiffer by threading it through an endotracheal tube exchanger or Eschman stylet preloaded with an endotracheal tube.

Combining Anterograde Fiberoptic Bronchoscopy with a Retrograde Wire

You can take advantage of both techniques to make intubation easier and faster. First, place a 0.035 cm ga. 145 cm long retrograde wire through the cricothyroid membrane and advance it into the oropharynx as described above. Insert your fiberoptic inside your endotracheal tube, then thread the guidewire into the fiberoptic's suction channel until the wire exits the channel near the eyepiece. Pull the guidewire rigid as you advance the fiberoptic/tube combination into the trachea. Remove the wire from below and insert the fiberoptic deeper into the trachea. Pass your endotracheal tube over the fiberoptic, then verify placement by listening to breath sounds.

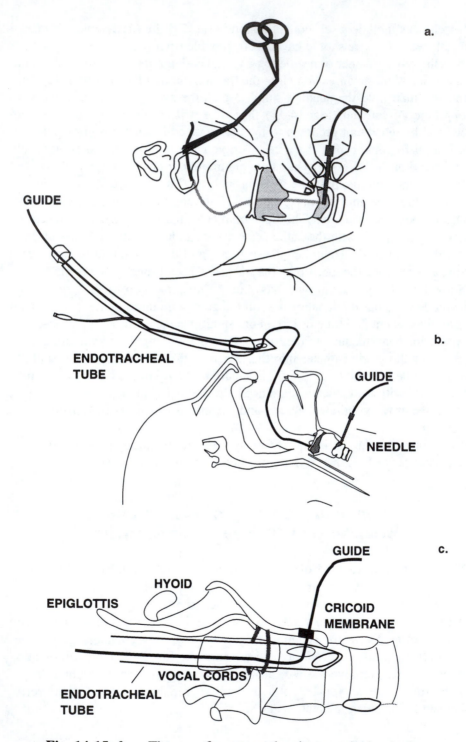

Fig. 14-15a,b,c. The use of a retrograde wire to assist intubation.

The Laryngeal Mask Airway as a Guide

The Laryngeal Mask Airway or LMA can be used either as a guide for blind intubaton or fiberoptic intubation. Ventilation can be performed during the procedure with the use of an angled endotracheal tube fiberoptic adaptor. This procedure is discussed in detail in Chapter 13.

Rigid Bronchoscopy

Intubation with a rigid bronchoscope sometimes works when all else fails. Improper use can cause severe trauma, so I don't recommend them for individuals not specifically trained in their use.

Further Reading

Carr RJ, Belani KG: Clinical assessment of the Augustine Guide for endotracheal intubation. *Anes Analg* 1994;78: 983-987

Dogra S, Falconer R, Latto IP: Successful difficult intubation. Tracheal tube placement over a gum-elastic bougie. *Anes* 1990; 45: 774-776.

Guggenberger H, Lenz G: Training in Retrograde Intubation. Correspondence. *Anes* 1988; 69:292.

Kovac AL: The Augustine Guide: a new device for blind orotracheal intubation. *Anesth Rev* XX:1; 1993: 25-29.

Lechman M, Donahoo J, MacVaugh H: Endotracheal Intubation Using Percutaneous Retrodrade Guidewire Insertion Follwed by Anterograde Fiberoptic Bronchoscopy. *Crit. Care. Med.* 1986; 14: 589-560

Nolan JP, Wilson ME: Endotracheal intubation in patients with potential cervical spine injuries.: An indication for the gum elastic-bougie. *Anes.* 1993; 49: 630-633.

Patil V, Stehling L, Zauder H: *Fiberoptic Endoscopy in Anesthesia.* Chicago-London. Year Book Medical Publishers.

15 AWAKE INTUBATION

G ood sedation reduces anxiety, speeds intubation, and often induces amnesia for a potentially unpleasant procedure. Local anesthesia also increases the comfort and ease of intubation. However, its use carries some risk.

Risks of Using Sedation

Under-sedation — Possible direct consequences include: poor cooperation raising the risk of trauma and aspiration; difficulty performing the intubation; hypertension and tachycardia; psychological trauma to the intubator; a poor evaluation of the medical care delivered.

Over-sedation — Over-sedation, however, can be more dangerous than under-sedation. Potential complications include: uncontrolled general anesthesia; hypoventilation (hypercarbia, hypoxia, apnea, cardiac arrest); decreased protective airway reflexes; aspiration; disorientation; poor cooperation.

Describing the intubation in *understandable* language reduces the need for sedation or anesthesia. Reassurance during intubation further reduces fear. "Hand holding" often works better than valium.

Learning to sedate properly takes practice. Always start with small doses and determine their effect before giving more. Table 15-1 lists common drugs and typical starting doses. Avoid the tendency to sedate heavily to make yourself feel more comfortable. As you gain skill you can often, *but not always*, predict the effect in advance.

We use two basic types of sedatives: hypnotics and analgesics. Hypnotics, such as valium, midazolam, or droperidol cause sleep and decrease anxiety. They often produce amnesia. Narcotics such as morphine, fentanyl, and demerol give analgesia, although they also add sedation. To treat anxiety, use a hypnotic. To treat pain, use a narcotic.

Table 15-1. Suggested Adult Starting Doses for Intravenous Sedation.

Drug	Intravenous Dosage	Advantages	Disadvantages/ Potential Side Effects
Valium (10mg/cc)	2.5-10 mg (0.035-0.15 mg/kg) give 1-2.5 mg increments	amnesia sedation minimal respiratory depression reversal with flumazenil	thrombophlebitis long acting no analgesia
Midazolam (1,5mg/cc)	1-5 mg (0.01-0.07mg/kg) give 0.5-1 mg increments	amnesia short acting (1-2 hrs) no active metabolites minimal respiratory depression reversal with flumazenil	no analgesia no reversal *6X stronger than valium*
Thiopental (25mg/cc)	25-75 mg (0.35-1 mg/kg) give 25-75 mg increments	amnesia very short acting (minutes) minimal respiratory depression *low dose*	antanalgesic hypotension disorientation reversal myocardial depression
Morphine (10 mg/cc)	1-5 mg (0.01-0.07 mg/kg) give 1-2 mg increments	good analgesia some sedation reversed with narcan	respiratory depression nausea / vomiting
Fentanyl (50 µg/cc)	25-75 µg *(microgram)* (0.35- 1 µg/kg) give 25 µg increments	good analgesia reversed with narcan	minimal sedation respiratory depression
Demerol (50 mg/cc)	12.5-50 mg (0.2- .75 mg/kg) give 12.5 mg increments	good analgesia reversed with narcan	respiratory depression nausea / vomiting tachycardia dry mouth
Droperidol (2.5 mg/cc)	1.25-5mg (0.02- 0.07 mg/kg) give 1.25 mg increments	sedation antiemetic	dysphoria
Ketamine (10, 50, 100 mg/cc)	10-100 mg give 10 mg increments	dissociative anesthetic (0.15- 1.5 mg/kg) active airway reflexes	hallucinations amnesia bronchodilator increased secretions tachycardia / hypertension increased intracranial pressure

Factors Influencing Drug Effect

Drug potency, dosage, route, and speed of administration — Giving larger doses or more potent drugs will increase sedation. Giving the medication very slowly reduces this effect. As a rule, intravenous drugs sedate more than intramuscular drugs, because levels in the brain rise more rapidly.

Previous drug exposure — Patients who drink heavily or who use narcotics or tranquilizers regularly need more sedation.

Pre-existing sedation — An already sedated patient needs less drug to lose consciousness. This is true even if he doesn't appear sleepy at the time. Potential causes for pre-existing sedation include:

- other drugs
- alcohol
- hypoxia
- hypoglycemia
- exhaustion
- hypothermia
- hyperthermia
- electrolyte or acid/base imbalances
- malnutrition
- shock
- hypercarbia

Age — Elderly patients and children need less drug for sedation.

Pre-existing disease — Renal or liver failure may alter metabolism or excretion of sedatives, increasing their effect.

Emotional state — Fear increases the tolerance for sedatives. Be careful, however. After the intubation the now calm patient may lose consciousness and become apneic. Sedatives also release inhibitions. A previously stoic patient may become uncooperative after a sedative.

Pain — Pain decreases the effectiveness of your sedatives. Once the discomfort is gone, the sedatives may suddenly take effect.

Diurnal rhythm — In my experience, it's easier to sedate patients at night than during the day. They often sleep longer once sedated.

Evaluating the Effect of Sedation

To judge the need for further sedation, evaluate the following.

Will the patient tolerate any sedation? Avoid sedation in shock, airway obstruction, or respiratory failure, unless it's absolutely necessary. These patients may become apneic, hypotensive, or obstruct their airways with small amounts of sedation.

Is this patient at risk for aspiration? Sedate lightly when there is risk of aspiration. Always have suction available and watch the patient.

Will sedation make the intubation safer? Patients with hypertension or angina need stress reduction. Struggling patients may injure themselves. Alert patients guard their airways more forcefully.

What is the emotional state of the patient? Calm, cooperative patients need little sedation. Fearful or belligerent patients may need a lot. Remember that hypoxia or hypotension cause restlessness and lack of cooperation. Rule these out before giving more sedation.

Is ventilation adequate? Check skin color, rate and depth of respirations, presence of breath sounds, and air exchange.

Careful medication and observation lets you use sedatives safely.

Local Anesthesia of the Oropharynx

Applying local anesthetics to the mucous membranes numbs them easily. However, such numbness is non-specific and hard to control. Injection of local anesthetics directly onto individual nerves anesthetizes quite specific areas of the pharynx and larynx. Such nerve blocks require knowledge of the anatomy and a recognition of the potential complications of each block. While I don't recommend them for the occasional intubator, they're valuable to the experienced intubator.

Internal Layngeal Nerve Block — The internal laryngeal nerve is a branch of the superior laryngeal nerve. It provides sensation over the laryngeal surface of the epiglottis, the larynx above the vocal cords, the vallecula, and the lower pharynx. It penetrates the thyro–hyoid membrane midway between the hyoid bone and the thyroid cartilage about 1 cm anterior to the superior thyroid cornu.

Pressing on the opposite side of the larynx makes the landmarks more obvious (Fig. 15-1). Clean the skin with antiseptic. Find the superior thryoid cornu

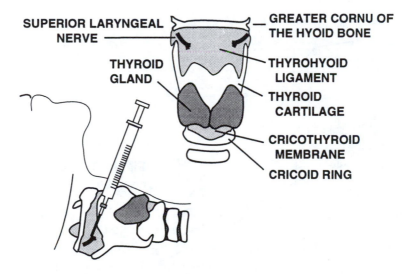

Fig. 15-1. Superior laryngeal nerve block.

on the block side. The carotid sheath lies beneath your finger and the internal la-ryngeal nerve lies in front of your fingertip. Insert a 25 or 26 g needle attached to a 3 cc syringe into the thyro–hyoid membrane. You will feel resistance when you enter the membrane at a depth of 1-2 cm. Inject 2 cc of 1-2% lidocaine at this point. If you can't feel the membrane, advance into the hypopharynx and as-pirate air. Withdraw the needle slowly until you can no longer aspirate air. Your needle tip should now lie just inside the membrane. Aspirate before you inject to avoid intravascular injections.

A block here preserves motor control of the cricothyroid muscle.

To avoid injection, place small sponges or gauzes soaked in 2% lidocaine into the piriform fossae bilaterally for 3-5 minutes. *Don't forget to remove them.*

Glossopharyngeal Nerve Block — The glossopharyngeal nerve gives sensa-tion to the posterior third of the tongue, uvula, soft palate, and the rest of the pharynx. A glossopharyngeal block lets you insert an oral airway within about one minute without causing the patient to gag.

Although you can use a 22 g spinal needle to perform the block, a 23 g ton-sillar needle makes the block easier and somewhat safer (Fig. 15-2). Depress the tongue with a tongue blade to stretch posterior tonsillar pillars. Insert the needle about 0.5 cm behind the midpoint of the posterior tonsillar pillar. Direct the tip laterally and posteriorly to a depth of 0.5-1cm. Aspirate carefully to avoid the carotid artery. A tonsillar needle has an angulated tip smaller than the rest of the needle to prevent deep insertion. Inject 3 cc 1% lidocaine bilaterally.

Combined internal laryngeal and glossopharyngeal blocks give excellent la-ryngeal anesthesia and depress the gag reflex. You may *cautiously* use them on patients with full stomachs because they preserve motor function. They pre-

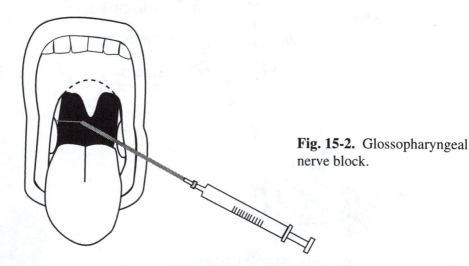

Fig. 15-2. Glossopharyngeal nerve block.

serve sensation below the vocal cords so any secretions or blood falling on or below the cords will still stimulate coughing.

Transtracheal Block — Transtracheal block provides anesthesia of the vocal cords, the subglottic larynx, and the trachea.

Insert a 23 g needle attached to a 3 cc syringe through the cricothyroid membrane (Fig. 15-3) and aspirate air to check placement. Hold the needle firmly in your non-dominant hand and the syringe in your dominant hand. Inject 2 cc of 1-2% lidocaine rapidly and then quickly remove the needle. The patient will cough. Some operators use 25-26 g needles. However, slower injection through the smaller needle means holding the needle firmly in place while the patient coughs.

A full stomach is a relative contraindication to transtracheal block. Maintain sensation below the vocal cords in this group if possible.

Acorn Nebulizers — Acorn nebulizers aerosolyze medications into the oropharynx and lungs, depositing a fine spray of droplets onto the mucous membranes and larger airways. We frequently use this device to treat bronchospasm. Aerosolyzing lidocaine will numb the entire oropharynx without injections.

Place 3-5 cc of 1-2% lidocaine into the nebulizer. Attach the nebulizer to your oxygen delivery system, such as a face mask. Wait until the liquid disappears, usually 15-20 minutes. By this time the pharynx, larynx, and trachea of the patient will be numb.

Complications of Local Anesthesia — Potential complications of injections include intravascular injection, bleeding into the airway, hema-toma, spread of tumor, and infection — although the risk of these is very low. Avoid airway blocks in patients with bleeding tendencies, infection, or tumor in the area of the injection.

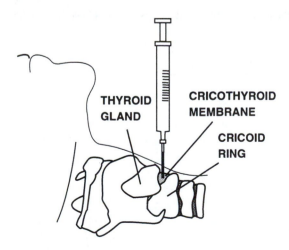

THYROID GLAND

CRICOTHYROID MEMBRANE

CRICOID RING

Fig. 15-3. Transtracheal nerve block.

Since oropharyngeal local anesthesia predisposes to aspiration guard against it. Always have suction available and use it frequently. Always suction the endotracheal tube after placement. *Never* leave the patient alone after numbing his airway, even if he seems awake and alert. Although aspiration can still occur despite all precautions, those precautions make it a very rare event.

Local anesthetic toxicity is a potentially serious problem. Calculate the cumulative total dose of local anesthetics *before* you use them. Don't give more than a total of 5 mg/kg of plain lidocaine or 7 mg/kg of lidocaine with epinephrine to your patient. Remember to add any local anesthetic needed elsewhere after the intubation.

Symptoms of local anesthetic toxicity are:

- sedation
- confusion
- tinnitus or ringing in ears
- apnea
- metallic taste
- loss of consciousness
- seizures
- arrythmias
- cardiac arrest
- heart block

Mucous membranes absorb medications rapidly. Don't let your patient swallow the local anesthetic. Instead, have him or her spit out the remaining liquid after holding the solutions in the mouth for several minutes.

If your patient shows signs of systemic toxicity then stop giving local, give oxygen, optimize airway and vital signs, and consider the use of valium to raise the local anesthetic seizure threshold.

Further Reading: Local Anesthesia

Barton S, Williams, D: Glossopharyngeal nerve block. *Arch. Otolaryng.* 1971; 93:186-188

Cooper M, Watson R: An improved regional anesthetic technique for peroral endoscopy. *Anes.* 1973; 43:372-374

Gaskill JR, Gillies DR: Local anesthesia for peroral endoscopy. *Arch. Otolaryng.* 1966; 84:654-657

16 INDUCTION AGENTS AND MUSCLE RELAXANTS

Seizures, agitation, and struggling can all impair the intubation process, causing poor visualization and difficult ventilation. Awake intubations can cause hypertension, tachycardia, increased intracranial pressure, and intense airway stimulation. This can cause certain patients — those with severe bronchospasm or head injury for instance — to decompensate. The use of sedative drugs to induce unconsiousness and the use of muscle relaxants to induce paralysis in these types of situations can result in an intubation that is easier to perform and safer for the patient.

While commonly used by anesthesia personnel, these drugs are gaining increasing use by emergency department physicians and, in some states, by paramedics. Their use requires special knowledge and training in the pharmacology of the drugs and the potential complications. Used correctly, these drugs can make intubation safer. Used incautiously, they can potentially cause injury or death. It's highly recommended that emergency departments contemplating use of these agents work closely with their anesthesia departments to establish protocols and quality assurance monitoring.

The use of induction agents and muscle relaxants to intubate by non-anesthesia personnel is still somewhat controversial and must be individualized to the patient. Moral support — combined with topical anesthesia — succeeds very well the majority of the time. However, there are times when it doesn't. The following discussion gives preliminary guidelines for the use of general anesthesia for intubation.

Preparing the Patient

Always have an assistant present. Preoxygenate the patient with 100% FiO_2 for several minutes if time allows. Have a means of ventilating the patient by mask ready for immediate use. Have suction ready, with both yankauer and flexible suction tips available and in easy reach.

Patients requiring emergency intubation are at high risk for aspiration. Have your assistant apply cricoid pressure and be prepared for vomiting. This assistant must hold cricoid pressure until told to release it after verification of tube placement in the trachea.

Monitor blood pressure and pulse rate closely. Pulse oximetry and EKG should also be monitored — if available — as desaturation and arrythmias can occur.

Most commonly used agents are short-lived and the patient will awaken within less than 10-15 minutes. Continued sedation will usually be needed to prevent hypertension or struggling due to the stimulation of the endotracheal tube. Have it on hand before you need it, then titrate accordingly.

Indications for Rapid Sequence Induction of Anesthesia

Rapid sequence induction is the administration of a sedative induction agent and a muscle relaxant to allow rapid placement of the endotracheal tube in such a way as to minimize change in vital signs and to avoid struggle. Cricoid pressure to avoid aspiration is usually held continuously from the time of administration of the drugs until the verification of proper tube placement in the trachea.

The use of purely awake intubation — using no sedation or muscle relaxant — is supposed to prevent aspiration. However, aspiration can occur in any patient, especially one with altered anatomy and airway reflexes. Insertion of the laryngoscope blade often causes gagging and interferes with protective reflexes. Muscle relaxants can speed the intubation process, reducing the time at risk for aspiration.

Awake intubation is supposed to minimize effects on the patient's cardiovascular system, and many times this is true. However, if a patient is fighting, a forced intubation will only worsen hypertension and tachycardia —which the older patient with a compromised cardiovascular system might not tolerate.

Intubating a struggling patient can traumatize the airway — breaking teeth, and causing laryngeal swelling and bleeding, among other complications. It can potentially worsen concurrent bronchospasm or cause laryngospasm. The struggle can also injure the intubator.

Sedatives and muscle relaxants can help when you can't intubate a patient easily or safely any other way. This may include the pediatric patient, or any patient with status epilepticus, severe bronchospasm, or increased intracranial pressure. The level of sedation can vary from a light dose promoting amnesia and calm, to a general anesthetic induction dose causing loss of consciousness. The choice depends on the patient's clinical situation and the experience of the intubator.

Tailoring the induction agent to the disease state is especially important because the choice of drug can either improve or worsen the symptoms. For example, the use of sodium pentothal in the patient with closed head injury can actually lower intracranial pressure (ICP). By contrast, ketamine, which can increase intracranial pressure and cause hypertension, should be avoided in the brain injured patient. Ketamine, on the other hand, causes bronchodilatation and is helpful in the asthmatic patient. Further discussion of the indications and contraindications of the various induction agents occurs later in this chapter.

Muscle relaxants themselves do *not* produce loss of consciousness or amnesia. They should rarely if ever be used without sedation in the conscious patient. Paralysis and intubation could be a horrifying experience in this patient — who would appear peacefully asleep to the health care provider. Serious hypertension, tachycardia, and possibly increased intracranial pressure could also occur. Muscle relaxants without some form of sedative should only be used in extreme emergencies, when the use of the sedative represents a greater risk to the patient than the failure to use one. Make sure that you continue to reassure the patient while they are paralyzed — even if you feel they are incapable of understanding you.

Relative Contraindications

The transient induction of unconsciousness can interfere with subsequent monitoring of mental status, because even the rapid acting drugs can sedate for several hours. Intravenous anesthetics can interact with whatever drug a patient has taken. They can also cause myocardiac depression, hypotension, and cardiovascular collapse in the hemodynamically unstable patient. If an induction agent is used in these patient groups you should adjust the dose accordingly and monitor the vital signs carefully. Any of these drugs can be fatal when used in the wrong circumstances and must be used with caution at all times.

Don't use induction agents or muscle relaxants if you're not skilled in both intubation *and* in ventilation with bag and mask apparatus. You must be trained in the management of complications encountered during the conduct of a general anesthetic. You *must* have manual ventilation equipment available *before* starting.

Avoid using muscle relaxants in any patient with airway obstruction. Muscle relaxation in these patients often makes obstruction worse as the intrinsic tone of the laryngeal muscles is lost along with the patient's own ability to ventilate. Avoid inducing unconsciousness in any patient who will be difficult to ventilate or intubate. Such patients include those with "smashed faces," morbidly obese individuals, and those with congenital anomalies such as Pierre-Robbin or Treacher Collins syndromes.

Use of Induction Agents

Sedatives used for emergency induction of anesthesia for intubation should optimally have rapid onset and short duration (see Table 16-1). All drugs used for induction of anesthesia must be given by or under the direction of a physician or anesthesia provider knowledgeable of the indications and contraindications of their use as well as skilled in airway management and ventilation.

Table 16-1. Suggested Doses for Induction of Unconsiousness.

Drug	Intravenous Dosage/Duration	Advantages	Disadvantages Potential Side Effects
Thiopental (25mg/cc)	1–5 mg/kg rapid onset lasts 10–20 min	lowers ICP anticonvulsant amnesia	hypotension myocardial depression respiratory depression antanalgesic no reversal
Ketamine	1–2 mg/kg onset rapid lasts 10–20 min	dissociative anesthetic bronchodilator (useful bronchospasm) transient rise BP and P (useful in shock) good analgesia	increased ICP tachycardia hypertension increased secretions active airway reflexes hallucinations (atropine reduces side effects)
Etomidate	0.2–0.6 mg/kg onset rapid lasts 5–20 min	hemodynamic stability amnesia	pain on injection seizure–like movements lowers serum cortisol high incidence n/v
Diazepam (10mg/cc)	2.5-10 mg onset 1–3 min lasts 5–20 min	amnesia anticonvulsant reversal with flumazenil	thrombophlebitis long acting sedation active metabolites no analgesia may cause hypotension
Midazolam	0.2–0.3 mg/kg onset 1–3 min lasts 20–45 min	amnesia anticonvulsant no active metabolites water soluble	hypotension possible

Intubation using an intravenous induction agent often requires a muscle relaxant to prevent patient movement during the attempt.

The barbiturate sodium thiopental, or pentothal, produces unconsiousness in less than 10-15 seconds after an intravenous dose of 2-4 mg/kg. This dose lasts 10-30 minutes depending upon patient status. When used in only sedative doses it can have anti-analgesic properties — increasing pain sensitivity and decreasing patient stoicism. Pentothal decreases intracranial pressure by causing cerebral vasoconstriction and decreased cerebral metabolic rate, making it very useful in brain injured patients. it also has anticonvulsant properties making it useful in seizures.

It does, however, have some disadvantages. It can produce serious hypotension due to peripheral vasodilatation and cardiac depression. You should therefore reduce the dose or use another drug in those patients with marginal cardiac reserve, hypovolemia, or shock. Pentothal can also exacerbate porphyria in those patients with that condition.

When pentothal is used in the patient with status asthmaticus, care must be taken to ensure that the patient is deeply anesthetized prior to placement of the tube. Bronchospasm may worsen as the result of stimulation during light anesthesia, *not* as a direct complication of pentothal.

Ketamine, a non-barbiturate anesthetic, produces rapid anesthesia, analgesia, and amnesia. Although it often maintains respirations and some degree of protective airway reflexes, the user should constantly guard the patient from aspiration and monitor adequate ventilation. A dose of 1-2 mg/kg induces anesthesia within one minute and lasts 10-15 minutes until start of wakeup. Concomitant use of a small dose of atropine or glycopyrrolate to avoid the common increase in oral secretions is highly recommended.

Ketamine's sympathomimetic stimulation tends to raise the blood pressure 10-50% above baseline and makes ketamine useful in the patient with hypovolemia or shock. It can, however, produce cardiac depression and in the patient who has exhausted his catecholemine stores it can produce hypotension like any of the other induction agents. Its ability to produce bronchodilation is useful in status asthmaticus.

Ketamine is relatively contraindicated in any patient who might be harmed by transient hypertension, such as the severe hypertensive, the patient with potentially increased intracranial pressure, or the patient with a leaking aneurysm. Use in these patients carries the risk of worsening their condition.

Ketamine can cause hallucinations, especially during emergence. Administration of diazepam or midazolam either early or late during ketamine anesthesia can counteract this effect. Maintenance of a quiet, reassuring environment during recovery also prevents problems.

Etomidate is a hypnotic drug without analgesic properties. Induction dose ranges from 0.2-0.6 mg/kg although 0.3 mg/kg is adequate for most patients.

Unconsiousness occurs within one minute and recovery begins within 5 minutes, similar to pentothal. Heart rate, myocardial metabolism, cardiac output, peripheral and pulmonary circulation are little changed by the drug. This makes it useful in those with poor cardiac reserve — although hypotension is possible and lower doses should be titrated in patients at risk.

Injection of etomidate is sometimes painful, this being less frequent when larger veins are used. Transient muscle movements occur in about 32% of patients, being classified variously as myoclonic, tonic, or averting movements. These can be mild to moderate but may appear disturbing and seizure-like. Etomidate induction causes nausea and vomiting in 25—50% of patients. Use of etomidate is associated with decreased plasma cortisol levels. Increased mortality has been reported in mechanically ventilated patients receiving continuos etomidate sedation. Steroid replacement should be considered, especially in those with pre-existing adrenal suppression.

One of the older drugs in use is diazepam, a benzodiazepine. Diazepam has less potential for hypotension than thiopental but its onset is slower and it lasts much longer. In fact, due to its active metabolites, an induction with a large dose of diazepam in an elderly individual can cause sedation lasting hours to days. Its induction dose is highly variable. It has anticonvulsant properties and can be useful in status epilepticus.

Midazolam, a newer relative of diazepam, has a faster onset and is more potent. The induction dose is 0.2-0.3 mg/kg. Onset is within 1 to 3 minutes. Patients are usually awake and responsive 45 minutes after the induction. There are no active metabolites. Midazolam can cause hypotension, probably due to decreased systemic vascular resistence and decreased venous return. Reduce the dose in hypovolemia and hemodynamic instability.

The choice of induction agent can be based on the patient's medical problem and hemodynamic stability (see Table 16-2).

Pharmacology of Muscle Relaxants

Muscle relaxants, or neuromuscular blockers, are medications which produce temporary paralysis of all the patient's muscles. They are commonly used in combination with general anesthetic induction drugs to allow rapid intubation as well as to produce a relaxed operative field during surgery.

There are two types of muscle relaxants: depolarizers like succinylcholine and nondepolarizers like vecuronium, atracurium, pancuronium, and d-tubocurarine. In an emergency situation we usually want a drug which will work fast and not last long, such as succinylcholine, vecuronium, or atracurium (see Table 16-3). As agents, panuronium and d-tubocurarine are so long acting in the emergency situation that they are often inappropriate for use in view of the shorter acting agents described in this chapter.

Table 16-2. Suggestions for Choice of Induction Agent.

Pathology/Stability	Agent
Head injury, hemodynamically stable	**high dose thiopental**
Head injury, mild hypotension or hypovolemia	**thiopental , decrease dosage**
Head injury, severe shock	**no sedative, or low dose thiopental, or etomidate**
Mild hypovotension/hypovolemia — no head injury	**ketamine or etomidate**
Severe hypovotension/hypovolemia — no head injury	**ketamine or etodmidate**
Status asthmaticus	**ketamine**
Poor myocardial reserve	**etomidate**

Table 16-3. Muscle Relaxants.

Drug	Intravenous Dosage/Duration	Advantages	Disadvantages Side Effects
succinylcholine	relaxation 1.5–2 mg/kg onset 1 min duration of effect: 5 min recovery time: 20 min	rapid onset short duration	increased intraocular P increased ICP tachycardia/bradycardia hypertension muscle pain hyperkalemia malignant hyperthermia
Vecuronium	defasciculation: 0.01mg/kg relaxation: 0.1 mg/kg for quicker onset: 0.15 mg/kg onset 2–3 min duration of effect: 30 min recovery time: 40–60 min	hemodynamic stability no dysrrythmia min cumulative effect	slower onset not for difficult airways longer duration
Atracurium	defasciculation: 0.05 mg/kg relaxation: 0.5 mg.kg onset 2–3 min duration of effect: 30 min recovery time: 40–60 min	liver/kidney failure shorter acting no cumulative effect	histamine release hypotension

Normal muscle contraction occurs when the electrical signal from the brain reaches the nerve ending and releases the neurotransmitter acetylcholine. Acetylcholine crosses the gap between the nerve ending and combines with the receptor at the neuromuscular junction on the muscle. This causes calcium to be released throughout the muscle. As a result, the muscle contracts. Acetylcholine is quickly removed from the receptor by breakdown by the enzyme pseudocholinesterase. Calcium returns to storage, and the muscle relaxes, ready for the next cycle. To use an anology, it is as though a key (acetylcholine) has entered the lock (or receptor) and then opened the lock (caused the muscle to contract). The key is then rapidly removed and the lock is ready to be opened once again.

Succinylcholine

A depolarizer like succinylcholine produces paralysis by combining with the same receptor that acetylcholine does. All the muscles in the body contract simultaneously. These massed contractions are called fasiculations. The muscles then become flaccid. The muscles remain paralyzed for many minutes because the enzyme pseudocholinesterase takes much longer to break down the drug than the natural neurotransmitter. In our analogy, the alternate key (succinylcholine) has entered and opened the lock (caused muscle contractions) but then becomes stuck for several minutes during which time the lock cannot be reopened (the muscle remains paralyzed).

Nondepolarizer type drugs, on the other hand, block the acetylcholine receptors but do not fire them, producing flaccid paralysis from their onset. Here our key enters the lock but cannot open it. However, the real key cannot open it either and the muscle remains paralyzed.

Succinylcholine is commonly used for emergency intubations because it takes effect within a minute and normally lasts less than 10 minutes. The use of succinylcholine is frequently preceded 1-3 minutes earlier by a tiny dose of nondepolarizer, such as 3 mg of curare or 0.5mg of Norcuron, to help decrease the strength of fasiculations and thereby prevent muscle soreness. Even this small dose can produce a decrease in respiratory reserve, especially in elderly patients. Monitor the patient carefully during this period.

The dose of succinylcholine is 1.0-1.5mg/kg. The diaphragm will recover before the muscle relaxant has completely worn off. Therefore, you must continue to ventilate for at least 10 minutes after breathing resumes. Assess adequacy of tidal volume at this time before you allow the patient to breathe unassisted.

If the patient receives a dose greater than 7 mg/kg of succinylcholine, muscle blockade becomes prolonged and may last many hours.

Succinylcholine also causes prolonged (1-24 hour) muscle relaxation in patients with myasthenia gravis, pseudocholinesterase deficiency, organophosphate poisoning, severe liver failure, or in patients using the glaucoma eyedrops phospholine iodide or echothiophate. This prolonged muscle relaxation is not dangerous as long as it's recognized and appropriate respiratory support provided.

Succinylcholine has caused marked hyperkalemia and sudden cardiac arrest in patients with extensive muscle damage or denervation, such as that following spinal cord injury, anoxic brain injury, severe muscle injuries or burns, motor nerve injury or tentanus and, rarely, intra-abdominal sepsis. This reaction develops variably from 24 hrs to 2 weeks following the injury. Most practitioners avoid its use in acute extensive crush or burn injuries simply because the actual time of onset of increased risk is unknown. Succinylcholine can potentially cause vitreous leakage in patients with open globe eye injuries.

Succinylcholine can increase intracranial pressure 5 to 10 mmHg, peaking within 3 minutes of drug administration. A small dose of non-depolarizing drug given to prevent fasciculations can help decrease this response and should be used whenever succinylcholine is given to the patient at risk. Intubating with a nondepolarizer is another option.

Succinylcholine can sometimes cause profound bradycardia, especially with repeat doses, or tachycardia. Monitor the pulse rate.

Malignant hyperthermia, an uncommon but potentially fatal hypermetabolic state, occurs in rare individuals. Athough this disorder is too complex to discuss here, signs which should raise concern are muscle rigidity — often heralded by masseter rigidity — unexplained tachycardia, metabolic acidosis, and hypercarbia. Fever, often rising in excess of 106°F or 41°C. If masseter or generalized persistant muscle rigidity is encountered after the use of succinylcholine, the drug should not be repeated and the patient must be monitored closely. Contact your department of anesthesia if you have any question because the expertise and the special medications to treat malignant hyperthermia will be there.

Because of the potential problems with succinylcholine, nondepolarizers are becoming more routine in the *hospital* setting. They should be used with great caution since their more prolonged action can cause problems if intubation is difficult.

Vecuronium

Vecuronium, a newer, shorter-acting, nondepolarizing agent with a dose of 0.1 mg/kg allows intubating conditions in 2-3 minutes. It lasts less than an hour, although it can often be pharmacologically reversed in 20-30 minutes. Higher doses of 0.15-0.2 mg/kg allow faster intubating conditions but last longer. Vecuronium has a roughly linear increase induration with increased dosage. As you double the dose you double the duration of effect. A good way to estimate its duration is to divide the total dose mcg/kg (micrograms/kg) by two.

Vecuronium doesn't cause bradycardia, tachycardia, hypertension, or hypotension and it avoids hyperkalemia in susceptible patients. This may be the agent of choice for those who need emergent intubation but can't receive succinylcholine. However, *don't* use any long-acting muscle relaxant if you have any question about your ability to ventilate or intubate. Guard against aspiration with cricoid pressure and suction as necessary. Be prepared to completely support ventilations during the intubation period and for several hours afterward.

Atracurium

Atracurium is also a nondepolarizer. It's dose is 0.5 mg/kg and it lasts from 30-60 minutes. Larger doses last longer, but do not have a cumulative effect. To estimate the approximate number of minutes of relaxation with atracurium, divide the dose in mcg/kg by ten.

Unlike vecuronium, atracurium isn't metabolized but undergoes Hoffman degradation of the molecule, self destructing independent of liver or kidney function. Unfortunately it has the tendency to produce histamine release in bolus doses, and thus has the potential for hypotension in patients prone to shock. This drop in blood pressure can be avoided with slow injection over one minute. Atracurium is the ideal drug for patients with liver or kidney disease.

Nondepolarizing muscle relaxants last longer than succinylcholine and will interfere with the ability to do serial neurologic exams for a prolonged period. You must reassure and perhaps sedate the conscious patient during this time to prevent undue anxiety.

Support respirations even if the patient continues to breathe until you are certain that the neuromuscular blockade is resolved.

Reversal of Muscle Relaxation

Neuromuscular blockade by muscle relaxants will eventually resolve spontaneously, although it may be prolonged in patients with severe liver or renal failure. However, there are many times when it is to the patient's advantage to have the neuromuscular blockade reversed. The end of a surgical procedure, preparation for weaning from the ventilator, and the need to follow neurologic exams are examples.

The drug class used to reverse neuromuscular blockade is called a cholinesterase inhibitor. These drugs temporarily inhibit the function of the enzyme pseudocholinesterase. This results in increased availability of the transmitter acetylcholine at the muscle end plate receptor. If sufficient time has passed for the concentration of the blocking agent to drop, then this flooding of the receptor with acetylcholine will allow the muscle to contract.

Only nondepolarizing type muscle relaxants such as vecuronium should be reversed. The use of reversal agents on routine succinlycholine blockade will *prolong* the block for many hours because the inhibition of pseudocholinesterase will also delay breakdown of the succinylcholine.

The dose used is either 0.035-0.07 mg/kg of neostigmine *or* 0.5-1 mg/kg of tensilon. Giving too much reversal agent will also cause paralysis because it then interferes with the natural neurotransmitter, acetylcholine, as well. If adequate reversal of neuromuscular blockade does not occur after the maximum reversal dose is given, then ventilate the patient until the blockade resolves on its own.

It's essential that the reversal agent always be given with either an equal volume of atropine *or* glycopyrrolate or serious bradycardia will result. The pulse rate should be monitored carefully for the next 10-20 minutes to ensure that late onset bradycardia does not occur. Use of glycopyrrolate, which has a longer half life, can help to prevent this side effect.

The patient should meet extubation criteria (Chapter 17) prior to removal of the endotracheal tube. Intact strength should be tested. The various tests have differing sensitivity for detecting residual muscle relaxation

The "Train of Four" setting on a peripheral nerve stimulator may return to baseline with 75% of receptors still blocked. Thus, the patient may not have adequate strength to cough or maintain their airway even though the test shows 100% function.

The "Tetanus" setting on a periferal nerve stimulator may return to baseline with 50% of receptors still blocked.

A heal lift can be sustained for 5 seconds or more only if less than 25% of the receptors are still blocked. This test is a simple and reliable method for testing strength, although abdominal pain and splinting of abdominal muscles may interfere with the patient's ability to cooperate.

You should always have the equipment readily available to ventilate or reintubate the patient prior to any extubation.

Further Reading

Yamamoto LG, Gregory KY, Britten AG: Rapid sequence anesthesia induction for emergency intubation. *Ped Emerg Care* : 1990; 6:200-213.

17 EXTUBATING AND EXCHANGING ENDOTRACHEAL TUBES

Removing an endotracheal tube is called extubation. Endotracheal tubes can be removed either because they are no longer needed or in order to exchange them for another endotracheal tube of different type or size. Both types of activities can have serious potential complications and must be approached with caution and preparation.

Extubation

Routine Extubation

Learning to intubate includes learning how and when to safely extubate a patient. Since endotracheal tubes are uncomfortable for the awake patient and can also cause trauma — especially with prolonged intubation — the endotracheal tube should be removed as soon as it is no longer needed. However, removing the tube too soon may predispose the patient to respiratory failure or airway obstruction requiring urgent re-intubation, which carries its own risks.

Carefully evaluate the patient prior to extubation. Criteria for extubation include:

- recovery of airway reflexes and response to command;
- no hypoxia, hypercarbia, or major acid/base imbalance;
- no cardiopulmonary instability;
- inspiratory capacity of at least 15 ml/kg;
- signs of intact muscle power;
- absence of retraction during spontaneous respiration;
- absence of a distended stomach;

In other words, you want your patient to be stable, able to breathe without help, and able to protect the airway.

Always suction the pharynx well prior to extubation because oral secretions drain into the trachea when you deflate the cuff. Also suction the endotracheal tube if there are secretions in it. Oxygenate the patient both before and after you suction the tube. Limit the time spent suctioning the tube to less than 10 seconds to prevent hypoxia. Make multiple passes if you have to clear a lot of secretions and oxygenate between each pass.

After you have suctioned and oxygenated the patient, untape the tube. Have the patient take a deep breath or manually assist the patient to take a deep breath. Deflate the cuff, and then pull the tube out quickly. The order of steps is important. If the lungs are already inflated, then the initial gas flow is outward. Frequently this will blow any secretions sticking to the cuff into the mouth where you can suction them. Squeezing the ventilation bag at the moment of extubation also helps blow secretions out. Deflation of the cuff should immediately precede extubation for the same reason — to prevent aspiration around the tube.

There is a high risk of laryngospasm and vomiting following extubation. Extubation during inspiration may have less risk. Have suction, oxygen, and the means to re-intubate the patient immediately available.

Extubating the Difficult Airway

Extubation of the patient with a difficult airway must be approached with caution. This is especially true if you expect the patient may be potentially difficult to ventilate. Removing the endotracheal tube too soon can predispose the patient to respiratory difficulties that the provider will find harder to treat.

If this is a fresh postoperative patient, it's usually best to wait until the patient is completely awake and able to breathe on his own.

A more challenging type of patient is one who has had airway edema from trauma or infection, which is now felt to be resolved enough for extubation to occur. Another is the patient with difficult airway anatomy and recent respiratory failure, who is now felt to have recovered sufficiently to no longer need assisted ventilation. Other examples include the patient in halo traction, or recovering from severe maxillo-facial trauma, or facial burns.

Begin by carefully assessing the patient by the criteria mentioned in the previous section. Are there any factors, such as continued infection or bleeding in the oropharynx, which might cause recurrent decompensation. If so, postponement of the extubation should be considered.

Extubating the patient at risk for respiratory failure or obstruction during the late evening or night shift, when nursing and physician staff is minimized, should be avoided if at all possible.

Plan ahead for the possibility that re-intubation may need to occur emergently. Have the equipment needed to proceed at the bedside. An emergency airway cart or "tackle" box serves well.

Optimally monitor the patient's pulse, blood pressure oxygen saturation. Have a knowledgeable assistant available to help. Tell the patient what you're going to do.

Consider the use of a device such as an endotracheal tube exchanger. The exchanger can be inserted down the endotracheal tube until it is between mid-trachea and carina. The endotracheal tube is removed over the top of it, leaving the exchanger in place as a possible guide for re-intubation if needed. Because a tube exchanger is hollow, oxygen can be insufflated or jet ventilated down the tube if the patient develops respiratory distress, averting a potential crisis situation.

The patient will usually tolerate the presence of the exchanger. You can assist this by injecting 50-100 mg of lidocaine down the endotracheal tube before inserting the exchanger and pulling the tube. Tape the exchanger at the corner of the mouth and note the depth.

Monitor the patient following extubation. Deciding when to remove the exchanger must be based on careful observation of the patient but you can typically remove it in about an hour if no problems have arisen.

You can extubate the patient over a bronchoscope under direct vision. However, leaving the bronchoscope in place as a guide should re-intubation need to occur is logistically cumbersome. It's heavy and must be held. There are no depth markings. It's expensive and the patient might bite it unless an oral airway or bite block is used. Finally, you're committed to reusing the same endotracheal tube. This may not be possible if edema has worsened following the extubation and may not be desirable it the tube is partially plugged with secretions. Finally, jet ventilating through a bronchoscope isn't optimal.

The American Society of Anesthesiologist's Task Force on Management of the Difficult Airway has published clinical practice guidelines for managing the difficult airway, including an extubation algorithm. These appears in Figure 17-1.

Re-Intubation Following Failed Extubation

Occasionally the patient fails the extubation attempt and requires re-intubation. You have optimally gathered all of your equipment together before the extubation in preparation for this potential event and can now proceed.

If you have a tube exchanger in position, you can either use it as a guide immediately or attempt conventional intubation first. If conventional intubation fails then the exchanger becomes plan "B."

To use the tube exchanger, slide the endotracheal tube down over it into the naso- or oropharynx. Consider the use of a tube smaller than the original to ease passage. Rotate the tube 90° so that the bevel faces posteriorly.

Have one of your assistants monitor the status of the patient and update you

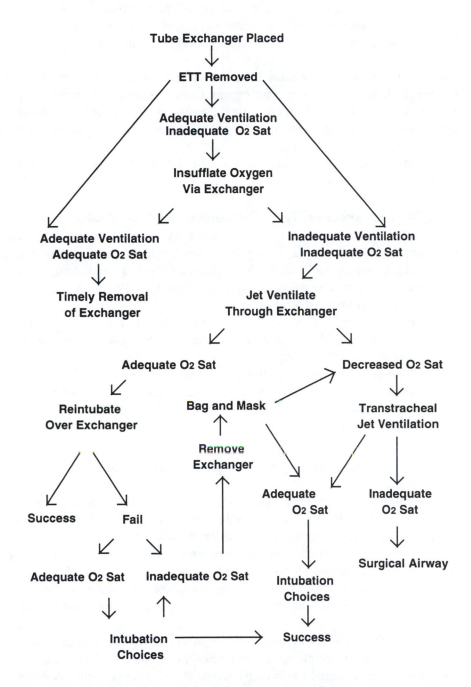

Fig. 17-1. Adapted from the American Society of Anesthesiologist's Task Force on Management of the Difficult Airway guidelines for managing the difficult airway, including an extubation algorithm.

regularly. Give oxygen. If you have a tube exchanger in place use it to provide oxygen. While you can simply insufflate oxygen down the exchanger, you will have to attach a jet ventilator if you need to ventilate the patient. See the next section.

If ventilation or oxygenation becomes difficult and there is no tube exchanger in place, apply higher concentrations of oxygen via face mask and positive pressure ventilation. If this fails then transtracheal jet ventilation should be considered if a "can't intubate, can't ventilate" situation ensues and hypoxemia is significant.

If intubation attempts continue to fail, you may need to consider a surgical airway.

Using the Endotracheal Tube Exchanger to Jet Ventilate

You can use a variety of adapters to connect your jet ventilator to an endotracheal tube exchanger, such as a 14 g IV catheter, a needleless IV port adapter, or a stopcock — preferably with a luer lock. Don't try to ventilate through the tube exchanger with a ventilation bag because you won't be able to generate enough air flow to inflate the lungs.

You usually need 20-25 psi to jet ventilate the lungs. You must keep the tip of the tube exchanger above the carina to minimize the risk of barotrauma and to allow ventilation of both lungs.

Watch the lungs inflate to an appropriate tidal volume and then allow enough time for them to deflate before inflating them again. As with any jet ventilation attempt, the airway above the jet must be open to allow unobstructed exhalation or pneumothorax will occur.

Changing an Endotracheal Tube

Sometimes it's necessary to exchange one endotracheal tube for another. Perhaps the cuff on the original tube is damaged and won't seal or a larger tube may be needed to allow bronchoscopy for examination or tracheal toilet.

If the airway is uncomplicated and there are no contraindications, the patient can have brief general anesthesia induced and the tube changed while they are asleep. The very ill or unstable patient may not tolerate this technique. If the airway is difficult, the possibility of losing the airway under deep anesthesia might be too great a risk.

There are several ways to approach this problem. The first is to make sure that the tube needs to be changed. Sometimes an endotracheal tube cuff which won't seal is not damaged but is above the cords. The signs of this problem are a cuff that won't seal despite injecting a lot of air into the balloon, a balloon which is tightly distended with air, and a tube which appears to be too shallow for the height of the patient. A chest Xray will often show the tip of the tube to be just below the larynx rather than mid-trachea.

If you suspect that this is occurring, make sure you have all the re-intubation equipment readily at hand just in case the tube slips out of the trachea. Then carefully untape the tube, suction the mouth, and insert the tube deeper into the trachea. Reseal the cuff and check immediately to make sure that the tube is still in the trachea and has not slipped into the esophagus.

If the tube needs to be changed, then the use of an endotracheal tube exchanger simplifies the procedure (Fig. 17-2). You can use it for both oral and nasal intubation. Optimally, attach an angled endotracheal tube adapter with a fiberoptic port to your endotracheal tube to allow continuous ventilation. Slide the tube exchanger down the tube through the port into the trachea until it lies just above the carina. You can inject 50-100 mg of lidocaine down the tube before you do this to improve patient comfort and tolerance. Tell the patient what you're about to do.

Once the exchanger is in position, suction the mouth well. Deflate the cuff and remove the original endotracheal tube by sliding it out over the top. Hold the exchanger firmly to prevent its backing out with the tube. Next, slide the new tube over the top of the exchanger and into the trachea. You will probably

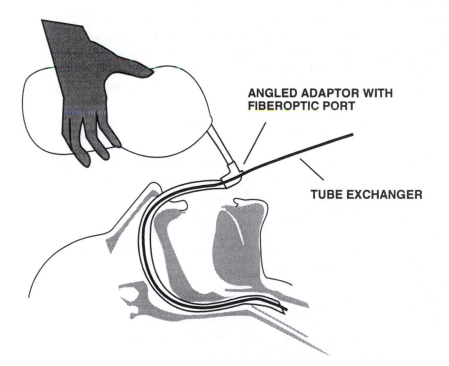

ANGLED ADAPTOR WITH FIBEROPTIC PORT

TUBE EXCHANGER

Fig. 17-2. Use of an endotracheal tube exchanger to change a tube.

have to rotate the bevel posteriorly to allow it to pass between the cords. Inflate the cuff, remove the exchanger and check immediately that the tube is in the trachea and not in the esophagus. If it's not in the trachea, you'll have to proceed immediately to alternative methods of intubation.

Alternatively, you can use a combined technique using a fiberoptic bronchoscope. Place your exchanger through an angled endotracheal tube adapter as described above and have your assistant continue to ventilate the patient. Load your new endotracheal tube onto your fiberoptic scope. Suction the mouth well. Deflate the cuff on the old tube and pass the fiberoptic through the mouth past the old tube into and down the trachea.

Once the fiberoptic is in the trachea, fix the fiberoptic in position. Have your assistant pull the old tube out, over the tube exchanger, leaving the exchanger in place. Pass the new endotracheal tube into the trachea. If all goes well and the new endotracheal tube is in the trachea, the tube exchanger can be removed. However, if the technique fails, then the tube exchanger can be used to ventilate the patient by jet until the next attempt can be made.

Further Reading

Benumof JL: Additional safety measures when changing endotracheal tubes. *Anes* 1991; 75:921-922

Benumof JL: Management of the difficult adult airway. *Anes* 1991; 75: 1087-1110

Caplan RA, Benumof JL, Berry FA: Practice guidelines for management of the difficult airway. A report by the Americal Society of Anesthesiologists Task Force on management of the difficult airway. *Anes* 1993; 78: 597-602

Miller KA, Harkin CP, Bailey PL: Postoperative tracheal intubation. *Anesth Analg* 1995; 80: 149-172

18 COMPLICATIONS

Any technique that we learn in medicine has potential complications. Fortunately, most complications are uncommon. Understanding the causes and routinely taking the steps to prevent them will ensure that they stay uncommon.

Complications from intubation can occur at any time — during the intubation procedure, while the patient remains intubated, or following the extubation (Table18-1).

Complications Occurring During the Intubation

Mechanical technique and the response of the patient cause the main problems that arise during the intubation. Trauma from excessive force or improper use of the laryngoscope blade can cause edema, bleeding, and damage to the teeth and soft tissue. Trauma frequently occurs in emergency situations when the intubator must hurry. Positioning is often less than optimal. Struggling in the conscious patient can prolong intubation attempts. The presence of a difficult airway also prolongs intubation.

Prolonged intubations predispose to the harmful physiologic responses of the patient listed in Table 12-1. Hypertension, arrhythmia, hypoxia, hypercapnia and respiratory acidosis, vomiting, and aspiration can all occur. Laryngospasm and bronchospasm from airway irritability or aspirated secretions happen more frequently. The intubator tends to become so fixated on the intubation that he or she forgets the patient. The temptation to interrupt CPR for longer than 15 seconds is great. It's also easy to forget to ventilate the patient between attempts and to suction the mouth.

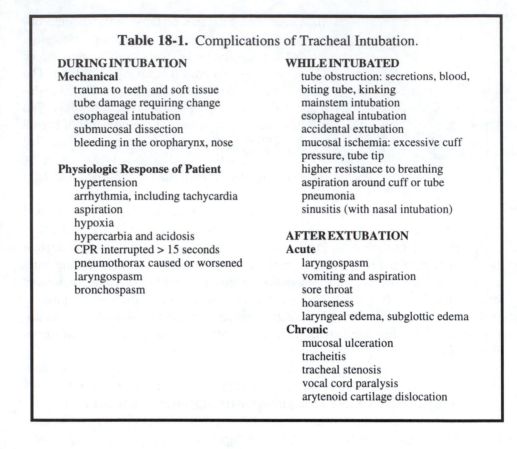

Table 18-1. Complications of Tracheal Intubation.

DURING INTUBATION
Mechanical
  trauma to teeth and soft tissue
  tube damage requiring change
  esophageal intubation
  submucosal dissection
  bleeding in the oropharynx, nose

Physiologic Response of Patient
  hypertension
  arrhythmia, including tachycardia
  aspiration
  hypoxia
  hypercarbia and acidosis
  CPR interrupted > 15 seconds
  pneumothorax caused or worsened
  laryngospasm
  bronchospasm

WHILE INTUBATED
  tube obstruction: secretions, blood,
  biting tube, kinking
  mainstem intubation
  esophageal intubation
  accidental extubation
  mucosal ischemia: excessive cuff
  pressure, tube tip
  higher resistance to breathing
  aspiration around cuff or tube
  pneumonia
  sinusitis (with nasal intubation)

AFTER EXTUBATION
Acute
  laryngospasm
  vomiting and aspiration
  sore throat
  hoarseness
  laryngeal edema, subglottic edema
Chronic
  mucosal ulceration
  tracheitis
  tracheal stenosis
  vocal cord paralysis
  arytenoid cartilage dislocation

The first step in preventing these complications is to place the care of the patient above the intubation itself. As long as you can ventilate the patient you have the time

- to do a gentle, purposeful intubation,
- to alter your technique and equipment,
- to reposition the patient, and
- to call for assistance.

You can *cautiously* sedate awake patients in the emergency situation — *being careful to avoid the loss of their respiratory drive or loss of their airway.* Treat hypertension and arrhythmia. Oxygenate and ventilate the patient between attempts. If you can't ventilate the patient then you shouldn't spend a long time on an intubation attempt.

Attention to the patient will slow you down a little bit. It will also keep your patient healthier. Because you're taking more time you will be less likely to traumatize.

Patients with irritable bronchi such as asthmatics or those with chronic obstructive pulmonary disease often develop bronchospasm, or wheezing. Topicalization of the trachea with 1% lidocaine — i.e., cardiac lidocaine 3-5 cc sprayed down the tube — may improve the patient's tolerance to the tube. The most common cause of wheezing in an intubated patient, however, is an endotracheal tube tip that either touches the carina or enters a bronchus. When you hear wheezing, check the depth of insertion and listen for the equality of breath sounds. Breath sounds may be equal if the tip is merely touching the carina. Try pulling the tube back slightly to see if this makes a difference. If the wheezing disappears you have your diagnosis. If it doesn't, treat the bronchospasm and get an X-ray as soon as you can.

If your patient vomits during the intubation attempt turn her on her side and quickly suction the pharynx. Place the bed in Trendelenburg if you can. Fast action can often prevent aspiration. Proceed with the intubation and immediately suction the endotracheal tube after you've placed it. Verify breath sounds. Wheezing, unequal breath sounds, an acidic pH. of the tracheal secretions, or actual vomitus or particulate matter in the endotracheal tube indicate a major aspiration. Aspirating as little as 0.4 ml/kg of pH 2.5 liquid can cause severe pneumonitis. Minor aspiration may remain asymptomatic. Treat major aspiration aggressively with bronchoscopy, tracheal toilet, and chest physiotherapy.

If the patient aspirates upon extubation you must use your clinical judgement as to the necessity of reintubation. Extubated patients are much better able to cough and deep breathe than intubated patients. On the other hand, applying positive inspiratory pressure or high concentrations of oxygen is much easier in the intubated patient. Let the patient's status be your guide.

Complications Occurring While Intubated

Mechanical problems with the endotracheal tube cause most of the complications during the period of intubation.

Patient movement will move the endotracheal tube. The tip of the tube follows the nose. If the nose points up, the tube rises in the larynx. If the nose points down, the tube descends. Extubation, esophageal intubation, and mainstem intubation can occur at any time. Nasal intubations minimize ascent or descent and thus are often preferred for long-standing intubations. Loose taping of the tube allows excessive movement.

Trauma to the trachea is the other major problem with movement of the tube. In fact, twisting of the tube can force its tip against the mucosa and cause ulceration. Secure the tube well to minimize the risk of trauma and misplacement. Avoid unnecessary patient movement. Use supports to prevent twisting of the tube.

Excessive inflation of the tube cuff also causes mucosal damage. Inflation to "minimal seal" and the use of pressure measuring devices can minimize this. Normally we inflate cuffs to 15 mmHg. This pressure usually prevents aspiration but is below the critical 25 mmHg pressure when mucosal ischemia starts to occur. Using the largest tube possible minimizes the cuff pressure needed to seal the trachea. This reduces the gap that the cuff must seal and therefore lowers the volume and pressure needed to do so. The cuff on the larger tube spreads the pressure more equally over the tracheal wall. The cuff on the smaller tube becomes rounded when distended and applies point pressure to the wall (Fig. 18-1).

Breathing through an endotracheal requires more force because the resistance is higher. This resistance increases in direct proportion to the length of the tube and to the *fourth* power of the radius of the tube. It makes sense that using the largest diameter tube will decrease this resistance. Weaning a respiratory cripple from a ventilator may depend on such small advantages.

Larger tubes also make the risk of obstruction less. They are far less likely to kink or plug with dried secretions or blood. Meticulous attention to tube positioning and cleansing of the tube will also prevent such dangerous obstructions. Allowing the patient to bite on the tube will also cause obstruction on occasion.

A final problem comes from infection. The larynx is a major barrier to infection. The endotracheal tube violates this barrier. Although sterile at the start of

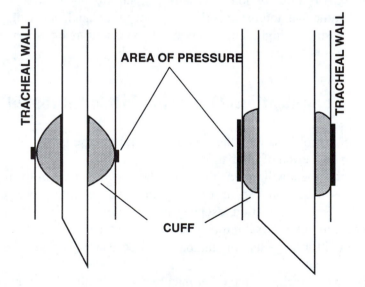

Fig. 18-1. Demonstration of cuff pressure distribution with different sized tubes. The wider the area of spread, the lower the pressure per square mm.

intubation, the endotracheal tube must pass through the mouth to enter the trachea. Bacteria can enter the lungs. Patients intubated for prolonged periods often have poorer oral hygiene. It's hard to brush your teeth with an endotracheal tube in place. Secretions passing the cuff and poor technique in suctioning the patient also allow bacteria to enter. In addition, intubated patients cough poorly. They can't close their glottis to generate the higher pressures needed to cough. Pneumonia can occur. Edema from minor tube trauma can cause obstruction of the sinuses and eustachian tubes, especially with nasal intubations. This predisposes to ear and sinus infections. Close attention to oral hygiene, careful asepsis, and frequent examination of the patient will help prevent infection.

Complications Following Extubation

Acute and chronic problems can follow extubation.

Laryngospasm usually occurs when the patient is only partially conscious at the moment of extubation. Extubation when the patient is still in stage 2 anesthesia, the excitement stage, is one example. In anesthesia we try to extubate patients either deeply anesthetized or totally awake — never in stage 2. At this time secretions or stimulation of the vocal cords causes reflex protective spasm. Unfortunately the rest of the brain is too asleep to turn it off. The patient may become hypoxic. Patients suffering from head trauma or heavy sedation are also at risk.

Treat laryngospasm with oxygen, positive pressure, and forceful upward pull on the jaw. Intravenous lidocaine 0.5-1 mg/kg sometimes helps. Only use muscle relaxants if you are experienced in their use. You can avoid laryngospasm by never extubating your patient partially awake, by carefully suctioning any secretions before extubation, and by being gentle.

Vomiting and aspiration can occur. Prepare for this with suction and heightened vigilance.

Minor edema often causes sore throats and hoarseness. Major edema causes airway obstruction. Young age predisposes the patient to problems simply because the small size of their airway makes even minor edema more important. Other predispositions include using too large a tube in a child, traumatic intubation, airway infection, and prolonged intubation. Tube trauma from excessive tube movement or an overinflated cuff can also cause problems.

Major edema of the larynx presents as post extubation croup. The patient, typically a child, develops a barking cough. The patient may have stridor or dyspnea. Conservative therapy consists of humidified oxygen by mask or a "croup tent" or treatment with aerosolized racemic epinephrine. This often shrinks the mucous membranes and resolves the obstruction. The dose of racemic epinephrine is 0.25 - 0.5 cc of 2.25% solution in 5 cc saline every 1-4 hours depending on the severity. Dexamethasone, 0.15 mg/kg may help prevent further edema formation. Severe cases may need reintubation. Croup can develop as long as 1-2 hours following extubation.

Tracheitis, tracheal stenosis, vocal cord paralysis, arytenoid cartilage dislocation all represent chronic complications. You can minimize the risk of the problems by the use of gentle technique and care throughout the patients intubation.

It is far better to prevent complications than to show skill in treating them. Forewarned is forearmed.

Further Reading

Byrum LJ, Pierce AK: Pulmonary aspiration of gastric contents. *Am. Rev. Respir. Dis.* 1976; 114: 1129

Harley HR: Laryngotracheal obstruction complicating tracheostomy or endotracheal intubation with assisted respiration. A Critical Review. *Thorax* 1971; 26: 493

Knowleson GTG, Bennett HFM: The pressures exerted on the trachea by endotracheal inflatable cuffs. *Br. J. Anaes.* 1970; 42: 834

Tarle DA, Chandler JE, Good JT, et.al.: Emergency room intubation — Complications and survival. *Chest* 1979; 75: 541

Vandam LD: Vomiting of gastric contents during the operative period. *N. Eng. J. Med.* 1965; 273: 1206

INDEX

Acid–Base balance: see pH
Acinus, 21
Acorn nebulizer, 209
Alveolus, 20, 21, 37
Alveolar Gas Equation, 28
Airway, anterior, 61–62, 132–133, 135
Airway, obstructed
  causes of, 18, 20, 40
  diagnosis of, 40–41, 42, 145–146, 148,
    158–160
  treatment of, 42–59
Airway, nasal:
  use of, 43, 47–48
  complication with, 48, 106
Airway, oral:
  use of, 43, 48–52
  complication with, 49, 106
Arytenoid cartilage, 15, 16
Aspiration:
  definition of, 12
  prevention of, 41, 108, 146–147, 185,
    204, 231
  treatment, 189–190
Atelectasis, 36
Atracurium, 217, 220
Augustine Guide, 190–194
Awake intubation: see Intubation, awake

B.A.A.M., 121
Bag, self–inflating, proper use of, 54–55
Bougie, 187–188
Breathing:
  work of, 21, 22–24, 43
Bronchi, 20–21
Bronchoscope, fiberoptic, 122, 152,
    194–200
Bronchoscope, rigid, 150
Carbon dioxide:
  diffusion, 22
  level in arterial blood, 25, 26, 27, 40
  retainer, 28, 29

Cervical spine injury, intubation and,
    136, 138, 148–152
Chest wall, 24
Children:
  anatomy of, 76y820, 24, 104–108
  choice of tube for, 110
  differences from adult, 104–108
  laryngoscopy in, 161–162
  respiration in, 34, 35, 107
Combitude, 177
Compliance, pulmonary, 58–59
CPR, intubation with, 125–129
Cricoid pressure, 16, 101, 109, 130, 140,
    141, 152
Cricothyroidotomy:
  needle, 177–178, 180–181
  surgical, 181–183
Cuffs, inflatable:
  proper inflation of, 70–71, 85
  complications with, 85, 232
  leaking, 70, 71
Cyanosis, 40, 41

Deadspace, 35
Diaphragm, 22–24, 38, 43
Diazepam, 214–216

Edema, 108, 233–234 (see also
    Intubation, fixed obstruction)
Edentulous patients, 54, 57–58, 97
Endotracheal tube:
  appropriate sizes, 82,110, 195
  checking of, 70–71
  depth of insertion of, 85–86, 99–100,
    102–103
  pediatric, 110
  securing of, 85–86, 87
Emphysema, 22, 29, 35
Epiglottitis,16,
  and intubation of children, 108–109

Esophageal intubation, accidental,
    100–101,111, 192
Esophageal Obturator Airway, 152 ,
    164–166,
Esophageal–Trachael Combitube,
    177–179
Etomidate, 214, 216
Extubation: 222–228
  criteria, 222–223
  difficult, 226

Fiberoptic: see Intubation, fiberoptic
Flexguide NCC, 186–187
Forceps, Magill, 68, 122
FRC: see Functional Residual Capacity
Functional Residual Capacity, 33–35, 38

Glascow Coma Score, 147

Hemoglobin, 31–33
Hgb: see hemoglobin
Howland lock, 189–190
Huffman prism, 190
Hypercarbia, 26, 27
Hyperventilation, 17, 26, 160
Hypocarbia, 27
Hypoventilation, 26, 28, 35, 39
Hypoxemia, 28, 30
Hypoxia, 28, 30, 39
  hypoxic drive and, 28
  signs of, 41

Induction agents (see also specific
    agents):
  choice of, 214–216, 217
  contraindications, 213–214
  use, 211–213
Infant: see Children
Intercostal muscles, 22
Intubation:
  awake, 196, 204–210, see also Chapter
    13
  burn victims, 158–159
  criteria, 38–40
  difficult:
    edentulous, 97, 132
    facial injuries, 159–160
    fiberoptic, 122, 152, 194–200

fixed obstruction, 136–139
head injury, 160
hemorrhage into airway, 140, 155–158
hypoxia during, 106, 184
in the field, 154–155
indications, 38–41, 147–148
LMA with, 174–176
mainstem, 101–102
neck immobility, 65, 133–136,
148–152
obesity, 60, 129, 131
overbite, 62, 133
receding chin, 61–62, 132
signs of, 63–67
laryngeal trauma, 160–161
nasotracheal:
  indications, 113–114, 150
  contraindications for, 66, 67, 114,
  150
  technique, 114–122
oral technique:
  blind, 121–122
  direct vision, 75–85
  tactile, 73
prevention of complications of, 184, see
  also Chapter 16
Ischemia, 27

Ketamine, 214, 215

Laryngeal Mask Airway, 152, 158,
    166–177
Laryngoscope:
  assembly of, 69–70
  preparation of, 69–70
Laryngoscope blade;
  curved vs straight, 70, 86, 89, 91, 92,
    131
  MacIntosh, 70, 78
  Miller, 70, 96–97
Laryngoscopy:
  direct, in adult, 75–85
  direct in children, 111–112
  positioning for, 76–78, 93–94, 110, 112
Laryngospasm, 18, 106–107, 229, 233
Larynx, 12–15, 17, 19, 65
Left handed intubators:
  laryngoscopy by, 94–95

Lightwand, 138
LTA, 185
Lung:
  anatomy, 20–22
  volumes, 33–35

Mallampati's signs, 63, 64
Masks, proper use of, 50, 52, 53–54
Midazolam, 214–216
Muscle relaxant:
  contraindication, 154
  definition, 216
  use, 153–154, 160, 216–221 (see also
    specific agents)
  reversal, 220–221

Narcotic, effect on respiration, 28
Nasal airway, 43, 47, 48
  ventilation with, 48
Neostigmine, 220–221
Nerve block,
  complications with,153, 207–210
    glossopharyngeal, 208
    internal laryngeal, 207–208
    transtracheal, 208–209
Nosebleed, 48

Obese patients, 23, 35, 56–57
Obstruction, fixed, 136, 139
Oxygen:
  content of blood, 25, 26, 29–32
  delivery, 29–33
  diffusion, 21–22, 36
  saturation, 30–31
Oxygen–Hemoglobin Dissociation
  Curve, 31

Packs, pharyngeal, use of with leaking
  cuff, 71
pH of blood, 25, 26–27, 40
Phrenic nerve, 22, 24
Pneumothorax, 35, 54
Polio blade, 187

Respiration, 22–24
  pediatric, 24

Safety, patient, 153, 184–185, see also
  Chapter 16
Sedation, 138, 145, 148, 153, 160,
  204–207
  dosages, 205
Shunt, pulmonary, 36
Sodium thiopental, 214–215
Stress, caregiver, 162
Stridor, 18, 41, 42, 43
Succinylcholine, 217, 218–219
Stylets, 71–72, 134, 135

Teeth:
  as cause of difficult intubation, 62, 63,
    97, 98
  protection of, 80, 97
Tensilon, 221
Thiopental: see sodium thiopental
Tidal volume, 33, 34, 35, 43
Thyroid cartilage, 13–15
Topical anesthesia, 116–117, 231
Toxicity, local anesthetic, 210
Trachea, 19– 20
  pediatric 20
Tube exchanger,122, 186, 224–227

Valium: see diazepam
Vecuronium, 219–220
Versed: see midazolam
Ventilation:
  causes of difficult, 23–24, 58–59
  technique, 34, 36, 37–38, 39, 50, 52,
    53–56, 58–59, 106–107
  in child, 24, 106–107
  in obese patient, 56–57
  in edentulous patient, 57–58
  in shock, 37–38, 40
  jet, 177–178, 179–180
  mismatch with perfusion, 37–38
Vocal cords, 15, 16, 17, 18, 19, 65–66
  paralysis, 18
V/Q mismatch: see ventilation, mismatch
Wire, retrograde, 200–202

ABOUT THE AUTHOR

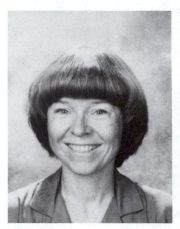

Dr. Christine E.Whitten is currently Chief of Anesthesia and Medical Director of Peri–operative Services at Kaiser Permanente Hospital in San Diego, California. She received her medical degree from Johns Hopkins Medical School in 1979. After her anesthesiology residency at the U.S. Naval Hospital in Portsmouth, Virginia, she completed fellowships in regional anesthesia and intensive care. Following training, she was on the teaching staff, Director of Regional Anesthesia, and Co-director of the Pain Clinic at the U.S. Naval Hospital in San Diego from 1983-1988. She became Board Certified in 1984.

Dr. Whitten is a co-author of "Anesthesia for the Developing Countries of the World" in *A Different Kind of Diplomacy: A Source Book for International Volunteers,* Plastic Surgery Research Foundation, San Diego, California, 1987. She is also the author of "Avoiding Anesthesia Mishaps in the 3rd World," *Seminars in Anesthesia,* "Third World Medicine Is an Excellent Model for Operational Medicine," *Military Medicine,* (Nov. 1988), a series of 11 articles on intubation and airway management in *Emergency Medicine*, and author of two teaching video series, one on perioperative nursing and a second on intubation and airway management. She has lectured before the California Society of Anesthesia, the California Association of Nurse Anesthetists, and Medical faculties in Kenya, Vietnam, Colombia and Nicaragua.

Dr. Whitten is an active volunteer for the international plastic surgery teams Operation Smile, Norfolk, Virginia and Interface, San Diego, California. Both groups provide free surgery to children of less-developed countries. Besides participating in the surgical teams, she has also instructed anesthesia providers during these trips to Mexico, Vietnam, Honduras, Nicaragua, the Philippines, Colombia, and Kenya.

Books, Slides and Videos for Intubation & Airway Management

Call 1-800-450-2665 for Free Brochure

KW Publications offers a variety of resources for teaching intubation and airway management, including the **4th edition** of the book *Anyone Can Intubate*, five full-color videos, color graphics slides, and a teacher's guide. All feature a unique step-by-step approach to the skills of intubation — ideal for training programs for:

• EMT-Ps • Anesthesia Residents • Nurse Anesthetists • Critical Care • PAs
• Emergency Medicine Residents • Respiratory Therapists • RNs • ACLS

Videos use real patients, not mannequins. Each of the videos is $99.95 each unless otherwise noted.
These full-color videos were authored by Christine E. Whitten, M.D., Chief of Anesthesia, Kaiser Permanente, San Diego. Dr. Whitten demonstrates step-by-step the intubation and airway management techniques and instruments. Videos are in 1/2 inch VHS format.

Basic Intubation Video (17 min.) Techniques for intubating adult patients

Managing the Airway Video (14 min.) How to manage airways

Pediatric Airway Management and Intubation Video (19 min.)

Fiberoptic Intubation (20 minutes).

Nasotracheal Intubation (26 minutes).

Color Slide Program enlivens presentations: $89.95.
Slide program consists of 69 **color** graphics slides based on the illustrations in *Anyone Can Intubate,* but with additional text added. Slides can easily be used independently of the book for classroom use by the instructor.

Free Teacher's Guide lightens class prep time
Teacher's Guide is *free* to any institution that buys the videos, slides, or adopts the book as required reading for their students. The guide consists of chapter by chapter suggestions for presenting the material, K-style multiple choice tests. The tests are laid out for easy duplication for classroom use.

Third World Volunteers: Prevention of Anesthetic Mishaps Video (30 min.) & Booklet. $29.95, $19.95 to overseas volunteer groups. *F*or anesthesia residents and practitioners electing an overseas rotation or volunteering their anesthesia skills in Third World countries.

Perioperative Nursing Videos

The Use of Intraspinal Opiates (26 minutes). **$39.95**

Assessment of Patients Following General Anesthesia (38 minutes). **$39.95**

Order Form: see following pages

30-Day Money-back Guarantee

Phone orders: Call **toll-free 1-800-450-2665**. **FAX: 1**-619-271-1425. By mail: **KW Publications**, P.O.B 26455., San Diego CA 92196 **Terms:** Net 30. Master Card, Visa, Checks or Purchase Orders accepted. Canada, other countries: payable in $ U.S.

- - - - - - - - - - Order Form (Please Print) - - - - - - - - - -

___ *Anyone Can Intubate, 4th Ed.,* paper @ $19.95.

___ **Basic Intubation** video, @ $99.95

___ **Managing the Airway** video @ $99.95.

___ **Pediatric Intubation** video @ $99.95

___ **Fiberoptic Intubation** video @ $99.95

___ **Nasotracheal Intubation** video @ $99.95.

___ **Intubation Color Graphics Slides** @ $89.95

___ **Third World Volunteers: Prevention of Anes. Mishaps** video @ $29.95/19.95

___ Please send *free Teacher's Guide* with the order.

___ **Perioperative Nursing: The Use of Intraspinal Opiates** video @ $39.95

—— **Perioperative Nursing: Assessment of Patients Following General Anesthesia** video @ $39.95 each.

_____ **$ Total for order. Add Calif. sales tax if applicable. Shipping billed at cost for multiple orders.**

Bill to: _____ Attn: _____

Street _____ City: _____

State _____ Zip _____ Phone ( ) _____

Resale # (Calif. only)_____ Purchase Order No. _____

Course

Reseller (if applicable) Volunteer Group (if applicable)

Ship to: _____ Attn: _____

Street _____ City: _____

State _____ Zip _____ Phone ( ) _____

Ship: ___ Library rate ___ UPS ___ Bookrate